CERTIFICATION REVIEW FOR PHARMACY TECHNICIANS

NINTH EDITION

NOAH REIFMAN, R.Ph., MS

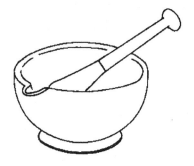

authorHOUSE®

AuthorHouse™
1663 Liberty Drive
Bloomington, IN 47403
www.authorhouse.com
Phone: 1-800-839-8640

First published by AuthorHouse 12/6/2011

ISBN: 978-1-4685-0730-0 (sc)
ISBN: 978-1-4685-0729-4 (e)

Printed in the United States of America

ABOUT THE AUTHOR

Noah Reifman, R.Ph.,M.S., a consulting pharmacist since1989, graduated from the Schwartz College of Pharmacy in 1980. He received his Masters from Temple University in Pharmacology/Toxicology. Noah has been involved in the education of pharmacy technicians for the past ten years in all areas of the ASHP Model Curriculum Competencies. He was the Director of the ASHP - Accredited Pharmacy Technician Program at Arapahoe Community College in Littleton, Colorado and was elected president of the Pharmacy Technician Educators Council (PTEC) in 2001. Noah has also authored a competency-based pharmaceutical mathematics text/workbook "MATH MASTER" PHARMACEUTICAL CALCULATIONS FOR THE ALLIED-HEALTH PROFESSIONAL (3rd edition). He also produced two educational videos on Reducing Medication Errors and Medication Administration. His interactive, online Certification Review Course was launched in 2006 (arkpharm.net).

Contibuting Author and Editor:
Jessica A. Trujillo, Pharm. D.

Enhance Your
PTCB Exam Success

Include our Online Certification Review Course and Pre-Testing Tools
Organized study plan
Key test-taking strategies
Proven learning techniques
Proven strategies for remarkable score-raising
Flexible study program that adapts to your study habits
Practice exams with evaluation of personalized strength/weaknesses

CONTENTS
- Six online review sessions covering all topics needed to excel on the exam.
- Math Master - Pharmaceutical Calculations" 3rd edition.
- Five Certification-like practice exams with online grading and strength/weakness trending.
- Post section "Proficiency Exams" assessing your progress.

arkpharm.net

Visit this LINK to purchase or take our free virtual tour of the course!

http://arkpharm.net/mspecials_onlinecourse.htm

By purchasing the new 9th edition of "Certification Review for Pharmacy Technicians", you are eligible for an upgrade to our interactive, online Certification Review Course.

TIPS ON TAKING THE CERTIFICATION EXAM

1) PLAY the percentages by eliminating as many wrong answers first and then deciding on a correct answer. This will increase your odds of answering the question correctly. With four possible correct answers, by eliminating two possible answers you have increased your odds from 1 in 4 to 1 in 2.

2) PACE yourself properly by first answering all the easy questions and then returning to tackle the hard ones. The National Certification Examination contains 100 multiple choice questions.

3) DON'T work so fast that you start making careless errors or too slowly that you are left with a shortage of time. You are given 2 hours to complete the National Certification Exam. To insure proper use of this time, bring an accurate watch to the exam in case the room does not have a clock.

4) ANSWER all questions on the exam. A blank space on your answer sheet is automatically considered a wrong answer, so even a random guess increases your odds and may ultimately increase your score.

5) CHANGE answers only if you have a reason for doing so. Last minute changes have been shown to have a negative effect on test scores.

6) BEWARE!! Most standardized exams stack harder questions in the beginning of the exam to possibly disturb the candidates concentration and psyche. If the first few questions seem overly difficult, skip over them and return to them at a later time. Remember that many times, future questions on an exam provide vital information for previous questions.

7) READ all answer choices before you decide on the correct answer. Watch out for answer choices designed to tempt the candidate into guessing incorrectly.

8) USE good judgement and best of luck.

TABLE OF CONTENTS

SECTION 2D: SAFE HANDLING OF ANTINEOPLASTIC DRUGS

SECTION 3: FEDERAL PHARMACY LAW

SECTION 4: MEDICAL, PHARMACEUTICAL TERMINOLOGY AND ABBREVIATIONS

SECTION 5: DRUG CLASSIFICATION

SECTION 7A: TASK EVALUATIONS - RETAIL

SECTION 7B: TASK EVALUATIONS - INSTITUTIONAL

SECTION 8: CERTIFICATION - TYPE QUESTIONS

SECTION 1: INTERPRETATION OF MEDICATION ORDERS AND PRESCRIPTIONS

A **DRUG** is a substance intended for use in the diagnosis, cure, treatment or prevention of disease in human beings or animals.

Drugs are available both by prescription and non-prescription.
1) **LEGEND DRUGS**
   a) refer to those medications that REQUIRE a prescription.
   b) "legend" refers to the phrase on every manufacturer's prescription drug stating "CAUTION: FEDERAL (USA) LAW PROHIBITS DISPENSING WITHOUT A PRESCRIPTION".
   c) not considered safe for use without medical supervision.
2) **OTC DRUGS**
   a) refer to those drugs that DO NOT REQUIRE a prescription.
   b) the letters OTC mean "OVER THE COUNTER" .
   c) considered safe for use without medical supervision.

THE PRESCRIPTION ORDER: "COMMUNITY PRACTICE"
A prescription is an order for a medication or medical device, issued by a licensed prescriber.
   a) licensed prescribers include the physician, dentist, veterinarian, podiatrist, physician's assistant and nurse practioners.
   b) Nurse Practioners and Physician's Assistants may also prescribe under the direct supervion of a licensed prescriber .
   c) only a licensed pharmacist or pharmacy intern may receive a telephone prescription from the above legal prescribers.
   d) pharmacy technicians may not transcribe telephone orders directly from the prescriber but may record authorized refill information including patient name and address, Rx number, date of original prescription, and pick-up or delivery times. This may change in the near future.

PARTS OF THE PRESCRIPTION ORDER:
1) PRESCRIBER INFORMATION
   a) name of prescriber must be imprinted on prescription order.
   b) address and phone of prescriber.
   c) Drug Enforcement Agency (DEA) number for controlled substances.
   d) State License number for certain 3rd party prescriptions.

2) PATIENT INFORMATION
   a) name and address of patient.
   b) age of patient.
   c) date the prescription was prescribed for the patient.

3) MEDICATION INFORMATION

    a) name, strength, dosage form, quantity and directions for use. This is referred to as the "dispensing directions".

    b) signature of prescriber indicating if BRAND or its GENERIC EQUIVALENT should be dispensed.

    c) indication as to the number of refills. If no refills are authorized, then the prescriber may indicate this fact by using the letters "NR".

BRAND, GENERIC, CHEMICAL NAMES:

1) BRAND or TRADE NAME

    a) designated by a superscript ® at the end of the drug name, indicating it has been registered with the US Patent Office.

    b) only the patent holder may use the trade/brand name of the drug.

    c) a brand name distinguishes a particular product from those of its competitors.

    d) if a brand drug is desired, the prescriber will indicate this fact by writing in the appropriate space "DAW", Dispense As Written.

2) GENERIC NAME

    a) is often a contraction of the chemical name, sometimes indicating the chemical class to which the drug belongs.

    b) if "DAW" is not indicated, then the generic equivalent will be dispensed.

    c) is properly referred to as its nonproprietary name.

3) CHEMICAL NAME

    a) describes the structure of the drug by standard chemical nomenclature.

GENERIC SUBSTITUTION:

   a) approved generic equivalents of brand name drugs may be substituted if the "DAW" is not indicated in the presciber's own handwriting.
   b) certain 3rd party payors require that the prescriber write on the prescription order "Brand Medically Necessary" for the brand drug to be dispensed, in addition to the "DAW" notation.
   c) generic drugs must be sold at a lower price than brand name drugs

PRESCRIPTION LABELING: (non-controlled drugs)

   1) LABEL REQUIREMENTS
      a) referred to as "dispensing labels" which must contain the following elements:
      - name, address and telephone number of pharmacy
      - prescription number
      - date of dispensing
      - patient name and address
      - name of medication
      - quantity of medication dispensed
      - directions for use
      - "auxiliary" or cautionary statements when applicable
      - prescriber's name

   2) AUXILIARY LABELS
      a) small labels that provide additional information, warnings, or reminders, that are affixed to the prescription container.
      b) care must be taken not to cover any part of the prescription label.
      c) information concerning proper use, handling, storage, or refill status.

DO NOT TAKE DAIRY PRODUCTS ANTACIDS OR IRON PREPARATIONS WITHIN ONE HOUR OF THIS MEDICATION	YOU SHOULD AVOID PROLONGED OR EXCESSIVE EXPOSURE TO DIRECT AND/OR ARTIFICIAL SUNLIGHT WHILE TAKING THIS MEDICATION	**DO NOT DRINK** ALCOHOLIC BEVERAGES WHEN TAKING THIS MEDICATION

PATIENT PROFILES:

The "patient medication profile" is a listing of all medications dispensed by the pharmacy to a particular patient. Patient information such as allergies, contraindications, and diagnosis allows the pharmacist to monitor for proper drug therapy. A complete patient profile should include but not be limited to the following information:

   a) name, address, and telephone number of individual patient or family.
   b) age and weight of patient.
   c) allergies - if there are no known allergies, then the letters "NKA" may be used to indicate this fact.
   d) contraindications to any medications.
   e) diagnosis
   f) 3rd party information.

REFILLS:
    1) NON-CONTROLLED DRUGS
        a) authorized refills must be indicated on the prescription.
        b) if no information regarding refills is indicated then it is assumed to be nonrefillable.
    2) CONTROLLED DRUGS
        a) see section on "CONTROLLED SUBSTANCES".

THE PRESCRIPTION ORDER: "INSTITUTIONAL PRACTICE"

Physicians orders for hospital inpatients or nursing home residents are written on "physician's order sheets". They may be hand written by the prescriber or computer generated with the physician's signature. It is common for these types of physicians orders to contain, in addition to medication orders, other instructions or patient care such as diet, therapy orders, required labs, and diagnosis.

LABELING:
    1) HOSPITAL INPATIENT LABELS
        a) since medications are administered by licensed nurses, pharmacy labels must contain the following patient information; name and location of patient, trade/generic name of drug, strength, and quantity. The unit-dosed drug will contain an expiration date and lot number on the packaged drug.
        b) injectable solutions must contain the name and concentration of each additive, the volume of IV solution, expiration date and time the admixture was prepared.
    2) NURSING HOME LABELS
        a) have the same labeling requirements as community practice since medication is not always administered by licensed nurses. Many residents in nursing homes self-administer medications or take their medications with them on home visits.
    3) HOSPITAL OUTPATIENT ORDERS
        a) have the same labeling requirements as community practice.

REPACKAGED MEDICATION LABELS:

Medications are commonly repackaged into unit-dose medications when either a specific dose is not commercially available or if bulk repackaging is cost effective. The pharmacy technician is usually directly involved in this activity and must be aware of the proper labeling and log keeping functions of this task.

    1) REPACKAGED LABELING
        a) each repackaged drug must contain a label that includes the following information: generic name of product, strength, drug dosage form, lot number, manufacturer's name, repackaging date, new expiration date of repackaged medication.

        b) anytime a brand drug is repacked, either in its original dosage form or is altered in strength i.e. broken in half on the manufacture's scored line, the drug is now considered a generic drug and must be labeled as such.

4

2) REPACKAGED LOG

    a) a "repackaging log" of all activities related to the repackaging process must be maintained and should include the following information; date of repackaging, name and strength of drug, manufacturer, lot number and original expiration date of drug and quantities repacked.

    b) each repackaged drug must be reviewed by a licensed pharmacist and indicated by a signature and date of review on the log.

PRESCRIPTION INTERPRETATION

The majority of prescriptions are written using Latin abbreviations. It is imperative that the pharmacy technician memorize each of these abbreviations and their meanings for proper prescription interpretation. Pharmaceutical Latin is used in pharmacy practice for the following reasons:

    a) acts as a common language for all pharmacists worldwide.

    b) provides a shorthand method for physicians to write prescriptions.

    c) reduces the possibility of tampering with the prescription.

COMMON LATIN ABBREVIATIONS:

ABBREVIATION	LATIN PHRASE	MEANING
a	ante	before
aa	ana	of each
ac	ante cibum	before meals
ad	ad	up to
ad lib	ad libitum	as much as desired
ad	aura dextro	right ear
as	aura sinister	left ear
am	ante meridian	before noon
au	aura utro	both ears
bid	bis in die	twice daily
c	cum	with
d	dentur	give
dtd	dentur talis	dispense of such doses
f, ft.	fac	make
gtt	gutta	drop
gtts	guttae	drops
h	hora	hour
hs	hora somni	at bedtime
M	misce	mix
M ft.	misce et fiat	mix + make
no	numus	number
noct	noctis	night

ABBREVIATION	LATIN PHRASE	MEANING
non rep, nr	non repetatur	no refills
od	oculo dextro	right eye
os	oculo sinsetra	left eye
ou	oculos utro	both eyes
p	post	after
pc	post cibum	after meals
per	per	by
po	per os	by mouth
pm	post meridian	after noon
pr	per rectum	rectally
prn	per re nata	as needed
q	quaque	every day
qod	—	every other day
q2h	quaque 2 horae	every 2 hours
q4h	quaque 4 horae	every 4 hours
qid	quarter per die	4 times daily
qs	quantum sufficiat	up to
qs ad	quantum sufficiat ad	add to the amount needed
Rx	recipe	you take
ss	semis	1/2
sig	signa	directions
sos	si opus sit	if needed
stat	statim	immediately
tid	ter in die	3 times daily
ut dict, ud	ut dictum	as directed

PHARMACEUTICAL DOSAGE FORMS

In actual pharmacy practice, pure drugs are seldom administered alone. They are combined with inactive materials (inert) to produce a pharmaceutical dosage form. The term "dosage form" refers to the physical form in which the drug product is made available for administration to the patient. The following section ill review the common dosage forms used in pharmacy practice today.

I) SOLID DOSAGE FORMS:

    1) TABLETS

        a) solid dosage forms prepared by mechanical compression in a tableting machine. Various formulation aids are added to the active ingredient such as diluents, excipients, binders, lubricants, disintegrators, coloring and flavoring agents.

        b) are the most popular dosage form in pharmacy practice and are available in various size, color, shape and weight. Some advantages are compactness, portability, accuracy, convenience and lack of taste.

        c) must be in its MOLECULAR FORM to be biologically active. This means the drug must first be dissolved in the stomach before it can elicit its pharmacological effect. This process is referred to as dissolution and is one reason why tablets have a relatively long onset of action.

2) CHEWABLE TABLETS
   a) compressed tablets that are designed to be chewed or dissolved in the mouth prior to swallowing.
   b) such tablets may be swallowed whole without chewing if a specific dose is required that is not available as non-chewable tablets.

3) ENTERIC-COATED TABLETS
   a) compressed tablets coated with special substances to prevent the dissolution within the stomach. These tablets are meant to dissolve in the intestines.
   b) these tablets may never be chewed, broken or crushed prior to ingestion. They also should not be taken with antacids since this causes dissolution in the stomach.

4) SUBLINGUAL TABLETS
   a) designed to be placed "under the tongue" where the active ingredient is promptly absorbed into the blood stream.
   b) only small amounts of drugs are required and absorption does not require the gastrointestinal tract.
   c) since it is absorbed under the tongue, it avoids the "first pass effect" in which the drug first circulates throughout the body before it is broken down in the liver (metabolized).

5) BUCCAL TABLETS
   a) designed to be placed "between gum and cheek" where the drug dissolves slowly over a period of time.

6) FILM-COATED TABLETS
   a) coated with a thin layer of water-soluble material that masks the objectionable odor or taste of certain medications.
   b) used commonly to protect sensitive drugs from deterioration due to light and air.

7) SUSTAINED, TIMED-RELEASE TABLETS
   a) special formulations where the active ingredient is released at a constant rate for a prolonged period of time (8-24 hours).
   b) commonly referred to as "long-acting", "delayed-release", or "prolonged-action" tablets.

8) LOZENGES
   a) also referred to as "troches or pastilles", which are solid dosage forms usually oval or discoid in shape.
   b) meant to dissolve slowly to keep the drug in contact with the mouth or throat for a prolonged period of time.

9) PELLETS
   a) small cylindrically shaped tablets meant for implantation subcutaneously (just under the skin) for prolonged continuous drug absorption.
   b) commonly used for such hormones as testosterone and estradiol and is currently being implanted as a method of birth control.

10) CAPSULES
   a) solid dosage forms in which the drug is enclosed within a soft or hard gelatin shell.
   b) after 10 to 30 minutes within the stomach, the gelatin capsule dissolves and the drug is released.
   c) sizes range from a number 000, the largest hard gelatin capsule commercially available, to a number 5 capsule, the smallest available.
   d) eliminates objectionable tastes and odors of certain drugs and are available in various distinguishable shapes and colors.

11) EFFERVESCENT TABLETS
   a) tablets containing, in addition to the active ingredient, sodium bicarbonate with either citric or tartaric acid. Upon dissolution in various solutions, the acid-base reaction causes "effervescence" by the liberation of carbon dioxide gas.
   b) serve to mask the taste of unpleasant, salty or bitter tasting medications.

II) LIQUID DOSAGE FORMS:

1) SOLUTIONS
   a) homogeneous mixtures containing one or more soluble ingredients (solute) dissolved usually in water (solvent), in which the molecules of solute are uniformly dispersed among those of the solvent.
   b) the solute may either be a liquid, solid or gas, while the solvent may be any water-miscible liquid. (hydrophilic = "hydro" meaning water and"philic" meaning loving).
   c) more quickly absorbed in the gastrointestinal (G.I.) tract because they do not have to undergo dissolution. They are also easier to swallow which may be necessary for pediatric or geriatric doses.
   d) both internal and external solutions are available and care must be given to clearly label external solutions "for external use only."

2) SYRUPS
   a) sweet, viscous, concentrated, aqueous solutions of sugar. It is used as a vehicle for antibiotics, antihistamines, antitussives (cough preparations) and vitamins as well as for other drugs.
   b) may be formulated with artificial sweetening agents for sugar restricted patients, i.e. diabetics.

3) ELIXIRS
   a) sweetened hydroalcoholic (water and alcohol) solutions and are probably the most widely used. Their popularity is due to their pleasant taste, relative stability and ease of preparation.

b) the concentration of alcohol may vary but usually contains no more than 20 percent alcohol. Alcohol is used because many drugs are more soluble in alcohol than in water.

4) TINCTURES
   a) alcoholic or hydroalcoholic solutions prepared from vegetable, animal or chemical materials. In general, tinctures contain a higher concentration of alcohol than do elixirs.

5) SUSPENSIONS
   a) preparations containing insoluble medicinal products (internal phase) dispersed in a liquid (external phase). The internal phase is generally in a very finely divided particle size. The external phase is usually aqueous containing a suitable flavoring agent.
   b) must be shaken well before use and care must be given to affix a "shake well" auxiliary label when dispensing this dosage form.
   c) among the preparations available are orally administered drugs, externally applied lotions and injectable medications.

6) EMULSIONS
   a) preparations containing either water dispersed in oil (w/o) or oil dispersed in water (o/w) stabilized with the aid of an "emulsifying agent". A third type of emulsion is called a microemulsion or transparent emulsion in which the particle size of the inner phase is 0.05 microns or less.
   b) both internal and external preparations are available and therefore must be labeled as such. Currently, intravenous fat emulsions are incorporated in Total Parenteral Nutritional (TPN) admixtures and will be discussed in more detail in the TPN section.
   c) as with suspensions, care must be given to label emulsions to properly shake well before each use.
   d) creams and ointments are emulsions in which the external phase is a semisolid.

III) TOPICAL DOSAGE FORMS:

1) OINTMENTS
   a) semisolid preparations used for external application to skin or mucous membranes. Besides serving as vehicles for topical application of medicinal agents, they also can function as emollients (lubricating agents) as well as protectants (prevent contact of the skin to irritants).
   b) ophthalmic ointments (eye) differ in that they must be sterile and be formulated for the special physiologic nature of the eye.
   c) requires a "For External Use Only" auxiliary label.

2) PASTES
   a) ointment-like preparations for external application. They are usually stiffer, less greasy and can pick up (absorb) more water than ointments.

b) frequently applied to oozing, weeping lesions because of their absorptive properties.

c) requires a "For External Use Only" auxiliary label.

3) CREAMS

a) semisolid emulsions, containing suspensions or solutions of medicinal agents intended for external application. They may either be water-in-oil

b) requires a "For External Use Only" auxiliary label.

4) POWDERS

a) finely divided, relatively dry, solid materials intended for external application.

b) certain powdered drugs are now available for inspiration into the lungs to help open the airways in patients who have asthma.

5) GELS and JELLIES

a) two phase systems consisting of a solid internal phase diffused through out a viscous liquid phase. The terms gels and jellies are used interchangeably.

b) requires a "For External Use Only" auxiliary label.

6) TRANSDERMAL PATCHES

a) patches applied to the skin formulated to deliver a constant, controlled dose of a medication through the skin and into the blood stream. The patch adheres to the skin by an adhesive layer on the outermost portion of the patch.

b) nitroglycerin, scopolamine, nicotine, estrogen and fentanyl patches are the most commonly used patches.

c) sites of application should be cleansed with alcohol and rotated. Repeated applications to the same site may cause irritation to the skin.

IV) OPHTHALMIC DOSAGE FORMS:

1) OPHTHALMIC DROPS

a) sterile solutions that are instilled into the eye in the form of an "eyedrop."

b) not an efficient dosage form because a majority of the eyedrop is squeezed out of the eye after blinking, making the time the drug is in contact with the eye extremely short.

c) since the eye can hold no more than 2 drops, patients instilling multiple medicated eyedrops should wait at least 5 minutes between instillations.

d) requires a "For The Eye" auxiliary label.

2) OPHTHALMIC OINTMENTS

a) sterile emulsions, properly formulated for application into the eye. This dosage form allows the medication to be in contact with the eye for a longer period of time.

b) upon application into the eye the patient's vision becomes blurred and is therefore recommended for bedtime use.

c) requires a "For The Eye" auxiliary label.

3) MEDICATED CONTACT LENSES

a) sterile contact lenses, pre-soaked with medication, inserted into the eye. This allows for controlled-release and prolonged contact of the drug with the eye.

b) now commercially available for certain antibiotics such as tetracycline and chloramphenicol. Contact lenses impregnated with pilocarpine, phenylephrine, and fluorescein are also available.

c) requires a "For The Eye" auxiliary label.

4) OCULAR INSERTS

a) drug pre-soaked inserts placed in the lower eye sac between the sclera (white of the eye) and the eyelid. This affords prolonged contact and controlled-released medication to the eye.

b) requires a "For The Eye" auxiliary label.

V) MISCELLANEOUS DOSAGE FORMS:

1) SUPPOSITORIES

a) solid dosage forms, usually medicated, for insertion into the rectum, vaginal cavity, or urethral tract. After insertion they melt or dissolve in the aqueous secretions of the cavity. Most suppositories exhibit their therapeutic effects locally while others are absorbed to produce a systemic effect (in the bloodstream).

b) adult rectal suppositories weigh approximately 2 grams and are usually 2.5 to 3.5 cm long. Pediatric suppositories are usually 1/2 the weight of adult suppositories or about 1 gram in weight. Vaginal suppositories are globular, ovoid or conical in shape and weigh 3 to 5 grams. Urethral suppositories are more slender, 3mm to 5mm in diameter and range in length from 60 to 75 mm for the female urethra, to 100 - 150 mm for the male urethra.

2) INHALERS

a) solutions or suspensions of solid or liquid particles in gas or air intended for inhalation via the nose or mouth. Only particle sizes of 0.5 to 3 microns will penetrate into the alveolar sacs within the lungs.

b) all inhalers must be shaken well before use and should contain a "Shake Well" auxiliary label.

3) OTIC PRODUCT

a) solutions or suspensions instilled into the ear canal. Larger volumes of medication may be instilled into the ear canal than in the eye and so 4 drops or more of an otic drop is not uncommon.

b) otic products should contain an auxiliary label "For The Ear" and "Shake Well" if it is a suspension.

4) ENEMAS

a) liquid medications introduced into the rectum via a bulb syringe. Their action can be either local or systemic and should be introduced into the rectum at room temperature.

5) DOUCHES
   a) aqueous solutions which are directed into a cavity of the body.
      Eye douches remove foreign particles or discharges from the
      eye, pharyngeal and nasal douches are used to cleanse or soothe
      the mucous membranes while vaginal douches cleanse and provide
      medication to the vaginal mucosa.

DOSAGE FORMS AND HOUSEHOLD TERMINOLOGY

DOSAGE FORM	HOUSEHOLD TERMINOLOGY
chewable tablets	chew, by mouth
external products	apply, externally
internal products	take, by mouth
inhalers:	
nasal	spray into nostril(s)
oral	inhale, by mouth
eye or ear products	instill into eye or ear
rectal products	insert, rectally
ocular inserts	insert into eye
transdermal patches	apply or place
vaginal products:	
creams	insert applicatorfull vaginally
tablets	insert tablet vaginally

LATIN ABBREVIATIONS - DOSAGE FORMS

ABBREVIATION	LATIN PHRASE	MEANING
cap	capsula	capsule
CR	—	controlled release
elix	elixir	elixir
EC	—	enteric-coated
ext	extractum	extract
fl	fluidus	fluid
LA	—	long-acting
soln	solutio	solution
SR	—	sustained release
supp	suppositorium	suppository
susp	suspensio	suspension
syr	syrupus	syrup
tab	tableta	tablet
tr	tinctura	tincture
ung	unguentum	ointment

UNIT DOSE DRUG DISTRIBUTION:

The fundamental elements to all unit-dose systems are:
1) medications are dispensed in single unit packages
2) medications are dispensed in ready to administer doses
3) only a 24 hour supply of medication is dispensed

Advantages of the unit-dose system are:
1) medication errors are reduced
2) control over medications is increased
3) drug waste and pilferage is minimized
4) nursing drug preparation and administration time is reduced
5) billing is more accurate
6) patient quality care is increased

The unit dose drug distribution system allows for less preparation time for nursing to administer medications and increased time for direct patient care. Patients are charged only for the medication they use because unit dosed drugs may be returned to stock and are not charged to the patient's account. Medication Administration Records (MAR) are provided by pharmacy to each nursing unit which allows for a coordinated and verifiable means of drug distribution. Unit dosed packaging allows for sealed, sanitary, accurate medications to be dispensed to the patient.

Types of unit dose distribution systems:
1) Centralized unit dose system - where the majority of medications are prepared and dispensed from one central location.
2) Decentralized unit dose system - where one or more "satellite" pharmacies are dispersed throughout the institution. This system allows for more interaction between pharmacy and direct care staff such as physicians, nurses and other health care professionals. However, the increased need for staff and inventory makes this system less cost effective.
3) Combination of the centralized and decentralized systems.

"**Coding**" refers to the notation on the medication order by the pharmacist or pharmacy technician of the name, strength and dosage form of the medication prepared for the patient. A pharmacist is required by law to review and interpret every medication order before any medication can be dispensed. All patient medications must also be checked by a licensed pharmacist before they can be dispensed to the patient. Medication profiles must be reviewed and checked by a pharmacist before any future orders can be filled.

Medications are dispensed to the patient in cassettes that fit directly into the nurse's medication administration cart. These cassettes must be exchanged on a daily basis to provide the patient with a complete supply of medication. The pharmacy technician is usually responsible for this function and must know which nursing units to deliver the cassettes and the proper times of exchange. When exchanging cassettes the pharmacy technician must remove any non-unit dosed medications from the old cassette and place them in the new restocked cassette.

An "Automatic stop order" refers to those medications that have a predesignated duration of therapy and must be discontinued if the physician has not reordered them. Automatic stop orders are determined by the Pharmacy and Therapeutics Committee and usually include such drugs as antibiotics, antineoplastic agents and other drugs that are not administered on a chronic basis.

PRODUCT NDC NUMBERS

All prescription medications are assigned National Drug Code (NDC) numbers by its manufacturer and must appear on each stock package. The NDC number is separated into 3 sections:
- a) section #1 - the first 5 digits identify the manufacturer of the drug product.
- b) section #2 - the 4 middle digits identify the product name, strength and dosage form.
- c) section #3 - the last 2 digits identify the package size.

example: 00029 - 6009 - 22

- a) 00029 - indicates the manufacturer is Beecham labs.
- b) 6009 - indicates the product is amoxicillin suspension 250mg/5ml.
- c) 22 - indicates the unit package size is 150ml.

EXPIRATION DATES

The expiration date of a medicinal product is the last date of sale as determined by the manufacturer. If the expiration date on a product states only the month and year (e.g., 3/15) then this infers that the drug expires the last day of that month (midnight 3/31/2015). Any sale of an expired product is considered unethical and is punishable by monetary penalties or greater.

PRACTICE PROBLEMS

PART I - PRESCRIPTION INTERPRETATION

Write the proper household directions for use on each of the following prescriptions:

1) i gtt ou bid x7d

2) i appl vag qhs

3) i tab po qid pc

4) iss tsp po tid prn cough

5) iv gtts ad q4h x5d

6) i supp pr q4h prn nausea

7) i cap po tid ac + hs

8) i tab sl prn chest pain

9) i tab po qod

10) ii stat, then i tab po qid x10d

11) Rx: Depakene syrup 250mg/5ml
      Sig: ii tsp po qid for 30 days
   a) What directions should appear on the prescription label?
   b) What quantity should be dispensed for this prescription?
   c) What is the total daily dose of this medication?

12) A prescription is written as follows: 1 tab qid x 1 day, 1 tab tid x 2 days, 1 tab bid x 3 days then 1 tab qd thereafter. How many tablets should be dispensed for a 30 day supply?

13) If a multi-dose vial is labeled 10mEq/ml and the following concentrations must be added to IV solutions: 20mEq/l for 3 liters, 25mEq/l for 3 liters and 30mEq/l for 2 liters. What is the total volume of drug needed to fill these orders?

14) Rx: Ceclor 250mg capsules
      Sig: 1 cap po tid x 10 days
   If patient is unable to swallow capsules, what volume of 250mg/5ml suspension should be dispensed?

15

15) Rx: Penicillin VK 250mg tabs
Sig: i gm stat then 0.5gm qid x10 days
a) How many tablets should be dispensed for this prescription?
b) What directions should appear on the dispensing label?

PART II - DOSAGE FORMS
Answer the following questions concerning pharmaceutical dosage forms:

1) Which dosage forms may never be crushed or chewed?

2) What would occur to a suspension if it was frozen accidentally?

3) Which dosage forms must always be shaken well prior to administration?

4) List examples of "parenteral" drug administration?

5) How is a "transdermal" drug administered?

PART III - AUXILIARY LABELS
Describe the proper auxiliary label(s) that should be affixed to the following drug products:

1) Pepcid suspension

2) Mycostatin Vag Tabs

3) Suprax 100mg/5ml suspension

4) MMR vaccine

5) Cortisporin Otic suspension

FOR COMPLETE ANSWERS
SEE NEXT PAGE

16

ANSWERS
PART I:

1) Instill one drop in each eye 2 times daily for 1 week

2) Insert one applicatorful vaginally every night at bedtime

3) Take one tablet by mouth 4 times daily after meals

4) Take 1+1/2 teaspoonsful (7.5ml) by mouth 3 times daily as needed for cough

5) Instill 4 drops into right ear every 4 hours for 5 days

6) Insert one suppository rectally every 4 hours as needed for nausea

7) Take one capsule by mouth 3 times daily before meals and at bedtime

8) Place one tablet under tongue when needed for chest pain

9) Take one tablet by mouth every other day

10) Take 2 tablets now, then one tablet by mouth 4 times daily for 10 days

11) a. Take 2 teaspoonsfuls (10ml) by mouth 4 times daily for 30 days
    b. 1200ml or 40 ounces   c. 2000mg or 2 grams

12) 40 tablets

13) 19.5ml

14) 15ml per day for 10 days = 150ml

15) a. 82 tablets for 40 total doses (4 times a day for 10 days = 40 doses). The first dose is 4 tabs while the remaining 39 doses are 2 tabs per dose for a total of 78 + 4 = 82 tablets. Remember that on day one, the first dose is 1 gm (4 tablets) and the remaining 3 doses are 500mg (2 tablets).
    b. Take 4 tablets now, then 2 tablets by mouth 4 times daily for 10 days

PART II:

1) Any controlled-released or enteric-coated medication must never be crushed or chewed. Controlled-released medications would deliver immediate multiple doses of a drug if crushed or chewed while enteric-coated medications would dissolve in the stomach rather than the intestine.

2) Refrigerator temperature is defined by the USP as between 2 and 8 degrees Centigrade or 36 and 46 degrees Fahrenheit. At times, a pharmacy refrigerator may exceed this range with products freezing. Suspensions that freeze may produce crystals but are redispersable upon shaking. Emulsions usually "crack" or separate upon freezing and are usually not redispersable.

3) All suspensions, emulsions and inhalant products must be shaken well prior to administration.

4) Parenteral drug administration includes: SC, IM and IV.

5) Transdermal medications are applied to and absorbed through the skin and are most often available as a patch. Patch sites must be rotated and patches should remain sealed until administration

PART III:

1) Shake Well, Expires 30 days after reconstitution. This preparation does not need refrigeration.

2) Refrigerate, For Vaginal Use

3) Shake Well, Discard after 14 days

4) Refrigerate

5) Shake Well, For the Ear

SECTION 2A: EXTEMPORANEOUS COMPOUNDING OF NON-STERILE PRODUCTS

The following section will review terminology, equipment, principles, and techniques involved with the extemporaneous preparation of non-sterile products. Even though the art of extemporaneous compounding has diminished due to the accessibility of a greater number of commercially available products, the need continues in the preparation of pediatric and geriatric dosages. It may be necessary to alter standard adult strengths and dosage forms for the pediatric and geriatric populations. There also remains a steady need for the preparation of dermatological products when combinations of various medications commonly prescribed by dermatologists are not commercially available.

WEIGHING refers to the determination of a definite weight of a material to be used in the compounding of a prescription or manufacturing of a dosage form. Weight is measured by means of a balance.

1) **BALANCES** = 3 types of balances are commonly used in pharmacy practice:

    a) *class A prescription balances* have a sensitivity requirement of 6 mg. This means that just 6 mg of a substance will move the pointer of the balance one division off equilibrium. Since only a 5% error is allowable when weighing substances, the minimum amount that may be weighed on a class A balance is 120 mg. The maximum weighable quantity is 120 grams. This type balance is required in every registered pharmacy by state boards of pharmacy.

    b) *bulk balances* are less accurate than class A balances and are primarily used for weighing large quantities of material.

    c) *digital balances* are sensitive to the tenth of a milligram and primarily used in place of class A balances in pharmacies.

Bulk Balance

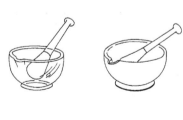

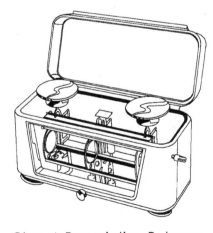

Class A Prescription Balance

Weights

2) **WEIGHTS** are usually made from brass or polished metal and must be maintained and handled properly to ensure accuracy. This includes the following recommendations:

    a) weights should never be touched by hand but rather manipulated with tweezers to prevent oxidation of the metal and the resultant inaccuracy of the weight.

    b) must be stored in a clean state, free of compounding materials and must never be dropped or dented, since this causes the weights to be inaccurate.

    c) once a year, the weights should be calibrated to ensure they are accurate. This is done by taking a properly calibrated set of weights and comparing these to the weights used in the pharmacy. Many pharmacy inspectors have documented the use of inaccurate, poorly kept weights used in current pharmacy practice.

3) **MORTARS** are bowl-shaped containers most frequently used in small scale trituration (grinding into a fine powder).
Three basic mortars are commonly used for compounding:

    a) *wedgewood mortars* have a rough surface making them well suited for grinding crystalline substances into fine powders. However, wedgewood is relatively porous and will stain quite easily and must be rinsed well after use to remove trapped substances.

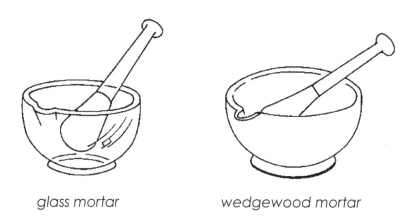

glass mortar   *wedgewood mortar*

    b) *glass mortars* are designed primarily for use in preparing solutions and suspensions of liquid materials. Glass has the advantage of being nonporous and not staining easily and is useful when flavoring oils or colored substances are used. Since glass is smooth it cannot be used for the trituration of hard solids. Glass also allows the compounder to view the contents and provides a visual means to evaluate if the solid has dissolved.

c) *porcelain mortars* are similar to wedgewood except that the external surface is glazed and is less porous than wedgewood. Porcelain should be used for the comminution of soft aggregates or crystals but is most commonly used for the blending of powders.

4) **PESTLES** (pes'tel) are instruments consisting of a handle and a rounded head that fits the shape of the interior surface of the mortar. They are made of the same material as the mortar and rely on proper contact between the head of the pestle and the interior surface of the mortar.

5) **SPATULAS** - 2 basic types of spatulas are commonly used. They are used to transfer solid ingredients from bottle to weighing pans, in the preparation of creams and ointments where they are pressed against the ointment slab in a back and forth motion to mix the ingredients and to loosen any powdered materials that have become packed onto the sides of a mortar during trituration. "Trituration" is the process whereby a mixture of fine powders is intimately mixed in a mortar. "Levigation" is the addition of a nonsolvent liquid to a powder to form a paste prior to the incorporation of a powder into a cream or ointment base.

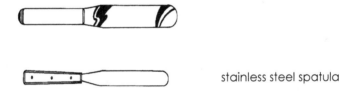

stainless steel spatula

a) *stainless steel spatulas* are flexible enough to bend and conform to the inner curve of the mortar. They aid in the removal of caked ingredients from the mortar and is the preferred spatula for the majority of compounds.

b) *hard rubber or plastic spatulas* are used to compound ingredients that react with metal such as iodine or the mercuric salts.

6) OINTMENT SLABS are flat surfaces of glass or nonabsorbable paper pads used to compound ointments or creams.

TECHNIQUES OF PROPER WEIGHING:

The pharmacy technician must know how to weigh out the ingredients for a compounded prescription. This includes proper technique and care for the class A prescription balance.
1) The position chosen for the balance should be a level and firm counter.
2) The scale must be balanced each time it is moved or its location is changed.

When properly balanced, the pointer should move an equal number of lines to the right and to the left of the center line. The pointer does not have to be stationary at the center line for the scale to be properly balanced.

3) Weighing papers on the left pan should be folded properly to insure no spillage when removing from pan. The proper folding pattern is to bring the lower left corner to upper right corner, forming 2 triangles. The procedure is followed from right to left, making the weighing paper more corrugated to hold more drug with less spillage.

4) The scale should be balanced with weighing papers on both pans.

5) Neither the weights nor any substance should be placed on the pans while the beam is free to oscillate.

6) The desired weight should be placed on the right pan while the substance to be weighed is placed on the left pan.

7) When adding or removing substances from the balance, always make sure that the lever is in the locked position. After addition or removal of a substance, the lever is turned to release the beam and the oscillations are observed.

8) The balance must be cleaned after use and stored in an area free of dampness, dust or corrosive vapors.

When mixing ingredients in a mortar, always place the drug with the smallest amount into the mortar first. Then add equal amounts of the remaining ingredients, mixing thoroughly between additions. Since the amount added to the mortar is equal to the amount in the mortar this process is known as GEOMETRIC DILUTION.

MEASURING OF LIQUIDS

Accurate measuring of liquids is an essential skill the pharmacy technician must learn and master. Equipment and technique used for proper measuring are contained in the following section.

1) **GRADUATES**

a) *conical graduates* are cone shaped measuring devices having a wide mouth slowly narrowing to its base. This graduate is mounted on a large circular base to prevent it from tipping over. As the diameter of the graduate increases its accuracy decreases but is used because liquids may be stirred in them and they are easy to clean.

b) *cylindrical graduates* have a uniform rather small diameter throughout the graduate and affords a greater degree of accuracy than the conical graduate.

conical   cylindrical

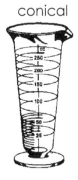
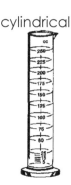

2) BEAKERS

a) cylindrical glass or plastic containers used for mixing of various liquids.
b) even though they are graduated and may be used for estimating volumes, they are not accurate enough for pharmaceutical measurements.

When measuring liquids in graduates, always choose the proper size graduate that is closest to the volume being measured. Avoid measurements of volumes below 20% of the graduated total capacity. For example, a 50 ml graduate will not accurately measure volumes below 10 ml.

Measurements should never be made in the unmarked portion of the graduate. For measurements below 20 ml it is often preferable to use a calibrated oral syringe.

Measurements should be made at eye level, always reading the bottom of the "meniscus". The meniscus is defined as the concave or semi-circle shape that the top portion of a liquid conforms to when in a graduated measuring device.

Graduates are either marked "TD" (to deliver) or "TC" (to contain). Graduates marked "TC" mean that the graduate will hold the desired volume but when transferred, a residual amount remains behind in the graduate making the volume measured slightly inaccurate. The "TD" indication means that the volume delivered from the graduate is the exact volume desired and the residual remaining solution is in addition to the volume measured.

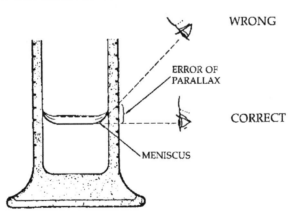

TECHNIQUE OF MEASURING LIQUIDS

1) the graduate is held at the bottom with the thumb and finger, using the pinky to support the underside.
2) the bottle is grasped with the right hand, label against the palm of the hand to prevent soiling the label.
3) the graduate is raised to eye level and the liquid is poured.
4) the liquid is poured until the bottom of the meniscus reaches the required mark.

RECONSTITUTION

Many oral liquids, especially antibiotics, are pharmaceutically prepared and stored in their powdered forms because they are more stable. Prior to use of the products, the proper amount of liquid must be added to powder to form a liquid. This is referred to as "reconstitution". Because the stability of the liquid is different than that of the powder, the new expiration date must be recalculated and indicated on the prescription label or an accompanying auxiliary label.

TECHNIQUES FOR RECONSTITUTION OF NONSTERILE ORAL POWDERS

1) measure the amount of "distilled water" or proper diluent as indicated on the manufacturer's label.
2) shake powder to loosen packed areas. This will aid in solubilizing the powder and will prevent packed areas from forming, especially at the bottom of the bottle.
3) add the required amount of diluent in divided portions as indicated on the label. Shake vigorously between additions.
4) if stock bottle, indicate date and time of reconstitution. Always indicate the new calculated expiration date on the product when dispensed and be sure to affix a "SHAKE WELL" auxiliary label if the product is a suspension.

SECTION 2B: PARENTERAL ADMIXTURES AND STERILE PRODUCTS

Parenteral products, which are defined as drugs administered via injection, have been estimated to account for greater than 40% of all drugs administered in institutional practice and for the majority of medications dispensed in homecare settings. It is therefore imperative that the pharmacy technician become familiar with all aspects of sterile product preparation, including equipment and technique. Aseptic technique which is defined as "a" = without, "sepsis" = fever causing organisms, refers to the preparation of a previously sterilized product without the introduction of microbacterial contamination.

The 3 major reasons why drugs are administered parenterally are:
a) the patient may not be able to take the drug orally because he/she is comatose, unconscious, nauseated, or vomiting.
b) a particular drug is not available in an oral form because many drugs are destroyed in the stomach.
c) an emergency situation may require immediate serum levels of a medication which can only be obtained via parenteral administration.

The major advantages of parenteral administration of drugs are:
a) the onset of action is more rapid than oral administration.
b) absorption into the bloodstream is more predictable than oral administration of a drug. Unlike orally administered medications, which first must undergo dissolution and absorption before the drug can get into to the bloodstream, parenterally administered drugs are absorbed rapidly and efficiently.

The major disadvantages of parenteral drug administration are:
a) the risk of infection when puncturing the skin with a contaminated needle.
b) unlike an oral drug where the drug can be removed by vomiting, adsorbed with charcoal or diluted if an error has been made after administration, parenterally administered medications are absorbed rapidly and are difficult to stop once administered.
c) parenteral drugs are associated with pain and psychological agitation.
d) the medication must be sterile prior to administration.

THE SYRINGE: The 2 basic parts of a syringe are:
a) barrel - a calibrated tube, tapered at one end to allow for the attachment of a needle. The open end contains a disc-shaped rim, to prevent the syringe from slipping between fingers. Needles may be attached by tight friction fitting or by a Luer-lock, which secures the needle with a threaded ring. For the manipulation of hazardous drugs, only a Luer-lock fitting may be used.

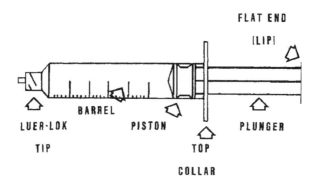

b) plunger - contains a lip or flat disc at one end and a cone-shaped rubber piston at the other end. The plunger must fit properly to allow free movement but must be snug enough to prevent the leakage of fluid from the syringe.

THE NEEDLE: The 2 basic parts of the needle are:
a) hub - is used to attach the needle to the syringe.
b) shaft - is usually metal and is coated with a sterile silicone coating for ease of insertion. Needle shafts should never be swabbed with alcohol or the coating will be destroyed. The tip of the needle shaft is beveled to form a point and is called the bevel tip. Needles must always be manipulated by their protective covers to prevent contamination.

NEEDLE SIZE: The size of a syringe needle is designated by 2 numbers:
a) gauge - diameter of needle bore and ranges from 27 to 13. Note that the larger the gauge, the smaller is the diameter of the bore. Therefore, 27 is the smallest available bore, while 13 represents the largest bore diameter.
b) length - measured in inches ranging from 3/8" to 3 1/2".

example: 10cc21G1" = the volume of the syringe is 10cc, the gauge of the needle is 21 and the length of the needle is 1 inch.

TRANSFER NEEDLES: Transfer needles are specially designed needles which look like 2 needles attached together at their hubs. They are used to transfer sterile solutions from one vial directly into another without the use of a syringe.

FILTER NEEDLES: Filter needles are needles which contain a filter near the hub of the needle. A 5 micron filter is the usual filter size, and is used to trap particles that fall into the solution. Filter needles should be used when opening ampules.

CORING: If a needle is inserted improperly through the rubber closure of a vial, pieces of rubber may be carved out as the needle is inserted and cause contamination of the parenteral product. This is referred to as "core formation". To avoid "coring", the following method should be used:
  a) lay the needle on the surface of the rubber closure so that the bevel of the needle is facing upwards.
  b) after inserting the bevel tip into the rubber closure, apply a slight lateral (sideways) and downward pressure to insert the remainder of the needle. When this technique is properly applied, the needle will curve slightly and core formation will be greatly reduced.

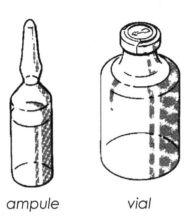

ampule   vial

VIALS: Vials of injectable medications are glass or plastic containers with rubber stoppers secured to its top by an aluminum band. This rubber stopper (diaphragm) is protected by an aluminum or flip-top plastic cover. Most protective caps do not guarantee sterility and therefore must be swabbed with isopropyl alcohol prior to needle insertion. Swabbing is accomplished with several wipes in the same direction over the rubber closure. The swabbing both disinfects and removes particles from the diaphragm. Allow time for top of vial to dry before puncturing with a needle.

Vials of medication represent closed-system containers since they do not allow for the equalization of either increased or decreased pressures. If air or a volume of solution is introduced into the vial, there is no passage out of this increased pressure and therefore pressure inside the vial is greater than outside of the vial. This is referred to as "positive pressure" inside the vial. In this instance, air or drug solution would prefer to leave the vial. If however, air or drug is removed from a closed-system vial, the pressure inside the vial would be lower than the pressure outside the vial and therefore air or drug solution would prefer to be drawn into the vial. This is referred to as "negative pressure" inside the vial or vacuum formation.

a) Hazardous drugs - it is important to maintain a slight negative pressure inside the vial. If positive pressure builds up inside the vial then hazardous drug solution may spray out and cause aerosol formation with possible exposure to the technician. With a slight negative pressure inside the vial, the tendency would be for the hazardous drug solution to be drawn inside the vial without contamination to the technician.

b) Non-hazardous drugs - inject a quantity of air into the vial equal to the volume of fluid to be removed from the vial.

AMPULES: Unlike vials, ampules consist entirely of glass once broken open, become open-system conainers and require no venting of positive or negative pressures. Ampules should be used once only and any unused contents should be discarded immediately.

a) Opening of ampules - the neck of the ampule is swabbed with an alcohol pad, leaving the pad in place after swabbing. The neck of the ampule has been marked with a "color-break" indicating where the glass has been weakened and can be easily and cleanly broken away. A firm snapping motion exerted away from oneself will cause the neck of the ampule to break. Never open an ampule towards the HEPA filter of a laminar flow hood.

b) Withdrawing medications from an ampule - tilt the ampule and place the tip of the syringe in the rounded area just below where the top has been removed. Surface tension should prevent the solution from spilling out during the removal of the drug.

c) Filtering ampule contents - to prevent the introduction of glass chips into an IV solution. Generally, the contents of the ampule are removed using a regular needle and then the needle is changed to a filter needle before pushing the drug out of the syringe.

ADMINISTRATION SETS: Administration sets consist of disposable, sterile tubing that connects the IV solution to the injection site. The solution container is "spiked" with the spike insert of the administration set and fluid travels directly into a drip chamber. A roll clamp, located below the drip chamber, allows for variable flow rate adjustment. A needle adapter is located at the opposite end with some administration sets containing y-site adapters and in-line filters.

I.V. SOLUTION CONTAINERS: IV solution containers are available in flexible PVC bags, semirigid polyolefin containers and glass containers. Each IV solution is carefully packaged to assure that the product remains free of any particulate or microbacterial contaminant.

a) large volume parenterals (LVP) are IV solutions packaged in glass or plastic containers holding 100ml or greater. Glass bottles are available with or without air tubes. Glass bottles without air tubes contain a vacuum and must be administered with an administration set containing a vent to allow air into the bottle as the solution is administered. The vent opening is covered by a bacterial retentive filter to reduce the intake of contaminated room air. Glass bottles with air tubes also contain a vacuum but there is no need for a vented administration set since the airway tube, which extends from the neck of the bottle to the bottom, allows for the equalization of pressure during administration. Plastic bags are also closed system containers with a vacuum. This allows for gradual collapse during administration without the need for venting.

Plastic bags are made from polyvinyl chloride (PVC) and contain two portals: an injection portal and an administration portal. The injection portal of a PVC bag contains two diaphragms, the inner approximately 3/8 inch below the outer, brown, latex diaphragm. Both diaphragms must be punctured for fluid transfer from the syringe. Therefore, a needle longer than 3/8 inch must be used for fluid transfers. The PVC bag offers the advantage of being unbreakable and lightweight, for easy storage.

ROUTES OF PARENTERAL ADMINISTRATION

ROUTE	ABBREVIATION	DEFINITION
intradermal	ID	"into the skin" Use short needle (3/8-5/8") with fine gauge (26G). Only very small volumes may be injected. Used for local anesthetics, diagnostic skin tests and desensitization of allergens. i.e. PPD
subcutaneous	SC, SQ	"under the skin" Use short needle (5/8") with fine gauge (26G). Usually not more than 2ml injected. Not for irritating drugs.
intramuscular	IM	"into the muscle" Use longer and larger gauge needles than SC. Preferred muscles are the deltoid (arm) and the gluteal (butt). Larger volumes of more irritating drug administered.
intravenous	IV	"into the vein"
intra-arterial	IA	"into the artery".
intracardiac	IC	"into the heart".
intrathecal	IT	"into spinal fluid"
intrasynovial		"into the joint"

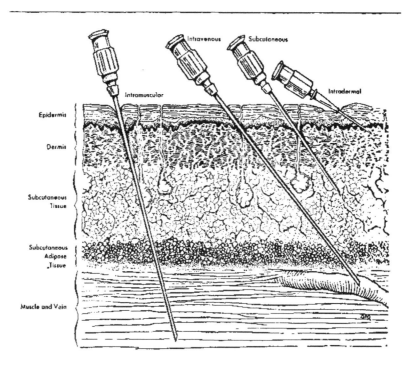

TYPES OF INTRAVENOUS MEDICATION ADMINISTRATION:

    a) **IV INJECTION** - also referred to as IV PUSH or IV BOLUS, is the administration of a relatively small volume of medication from a syringe over a short period of time.

    b) **IV INFUSION** - is the introduction of large volumes of fluids over long periods of time. Used commonly for dehydration, to restore depleted blood volume, to administer nutrients or to serve as the vehicle for medication administration. Two types of IV infusions administered are:

        i) Continuous Infusions or large volumes of fluids administered at a slow, constant rate over several hours. An example of this would be the administration of 1 liter of 0.9% NaCl over an 8 hour period, for rehydration.

        ii) Intermittent Infusions or relatively small volumes (25 to 100ml) of fluids administered over a short, specific interval of time. An example of this would be the administration of 50ml of 0.9% NaCl, containing 500mg of ampicillin, over a 15-30 minute interval every 6 hours. In this instance, rather than having to stick the patient prior to each administration (q6h x10days = 40 sticks), the intermittent infusion is "piggybacked" into the tubing of a continuous infusion, thus having two containers flowing into the patients vein through a common tubing and a common injection site. This is referred to as an "IVPB", intravenous piggyback. The IVPB must be hung slightly higher than the primary solution to allow the contents of the IVPB to flow through the injection site.

ADVANTAGES OF IVPB ADMINISTRATION:

  a) the patient will not have a catheter or needle inserted at each dosing interval.
  b) two medicatons may be administered at two different infusion rates.

VOLUME CONTROL SETS (BURETROL) Volume control sets are calibrated, plastic fluid chambers used to administer intermittent IV solutions in a precise manner. The buretrol is hung between the IV solution and the administration set permitting precise measurement of infused solution. Unstable drugs may be diluted in a minimum amount of solution and administered rapidly.

CHARACTERISTICS OF I.V. SOLUTIONS:

Intravenous solutions must possess certain characteristics in order to be infused directly into the vein. These qualities include:

  a) **clarity** - I.V. solutions must be clear. Solutions may be colored, for example adriamycin - red, MVI - yellow, but never cloudy. Fat emulsion for TPN administration, is one notable exception to this rule.

  b) **sterility** - Since the solution is introduced directly into the bloodstream, any microbacterial contamination found in the solution will also be directly introduced into the bloodstream. Therefore, all I.V. solutions must be sterile and remain sterile until the completion of administration.

  c) **pH** - the degree of acidity or basicity of a solution. The pH is related to the concentration of hydrogen ions (H+) in solution. pH values range from 0 to 14, with 0-7 being "acidic", 7 being neutral and above 7 being "basic" or "alkaline". Plasma, with a pH of 7.4, is slightly alkaline. I.V. solutions should be as close to neutral as possible. Extremely acidic or basic solutions will cause irritation and pain at the injection site.

  d) **isotonicity** - the physical phenomenon related to the number of solute particles in a solution. A solution that contains the same number of particles as blood is referred to as ISOTONIC. When a red blood cell (RBC) is placed in an isotonic solution, such as normal saline, no change occurs to the RBC. If a RBC is placed in a solution containing less particles than blood or HYPOTONIC, the RBC will swell since water will be pulled to an area of greater solute concentration (inside the RBC). If the RBC is placed in a solution containing a greater number of particles than blood or HYPERTONIC, the RBC will shrink since water will be pulled out of the RBC. I.V. solutions should be as close isotonic as possible to reduce patient discomfort and damage to red blood cells.

COMMONLY ADMINISTERED I.V. SOLUTIONS

I.V. SOLUTION	CONTENTS	TONICITY VALUE
D5W	5% dextrose	isotonic
D10W	10% dextrose	hypertonic
Normal Saline (NS)	0.9% NaCl	isotonic
1/2 NS	0.45% NaCl	hypotonic
1/4 NS	0.22% NaCl	hypotonic
D5/NS	5% dextrose + 0.9% NaCl	hypertonic
D5-1/2NS	5% dextrose + 0.45% NaCl	hypertonic
D5-1/4NS	5% dextrose + 0.22% NaCl	isotonic
Lactated Ringer's	Na, K, Ca, Cl, lactate	isotonic

INCOMPATIBILITIES OF I.V. ADMIXTURES:
An I.V. incompatibility may occur when the drug and the I.V. solution or multiple intravenous drugs are mixed within the same admixture and produce an undesirable change of those medications.

The three basic types of incompatibilities are:
   a) **physical incompatibilities** occur usually as a result of a change in solubility of a drug. A visual change occurs, such as a change in color, development of a milky haze or the formation of a precipitate. In many instances, the precipitate will not be evident immediately but may occur after refrigeration or upon standing. An example of this type of incompatibility is the mixing of calcium and phosphate salts in hyperalimentation solutions. A white precipitate is formed and the solution is rendered unusable.
   Remember, this type of incompatibility can be overcome by diluting each ingredient first and then mixing them with constant agitation. Phenobarbital (Pb) phenytoin (Dilantin) and diazepam (Valium) all have relatively low water solubilities and will precipitate out of solution if not mixed with a special propylene glycol diluent.
   b) **chemical incompatibilities** result from a chemical reaction between one or more elements of the I.V. admixture. In this type of incompatibility, no visual change may be noted and many of these incompatibilities go undetected. pH changes due to addition of highly acidic or alkaline drugs account for the majority of chemical incompatibilities. Decomposition of a drug by light is also a chemical incompatability and therefore solutions containing such drugs as nitroprusside or amphotericin B, must be wrapped in dark or tinfoil bags to protect the drug from light. The antimicrobial effects of ampicillin may be reduced when mixed with dextrose solutions or hydrocortisone sodium succinate.
   c) **therapeutic incompatibilities** result from the mixing together of two or more drugs which causes a change in the therapeutic response of one or both of the drugs. If penicillin is mixed with an aminoglycoside or a tetracycline, the antimicrobial effects of both these drugs will be diminished. Certain drugs will be adsorbed (bound to) or will cause damage to polyvinyl chloride (PVC) plastic bags and therefore must be dispensed in non-PVC containers and tubing. Insulin and nitroglycerin are examples of drugs that bind to PVC plastic while Taxol and teniposide tend to damage PVC plastics.

LAMINAR FLOW HOODS: Sterile products should be prepared in a "Class 100" environment, which is defined as containing no more than 100 particles, 5 microns or larger, per cubic foot. Since room air may contain thousands of suspended particles per cubic foot, laminar flow hoods are utilized to achieve a "Class 100" environment for the preparation of sterile products.

The 2 basic types of laminar flow hoods are:

a) **Horizontal Flow Hoods** - air is taken into the unit and passed through a prefilter, which removes gross contaminants such as dust and lint. The air is then compressed and distributed evenly through the "high efficiency particulate air" filter (HEPA) to create a constant air flow of approximately 90 linear feet per minute across the work surface. The HEPA filter, which is bacteria retentive, removes 99.9% of particles 0.3 microns or larger from the work surface, thereby removing nearly all bacteria. In horizontal hoods, the HEPA filter constitutes the entire back portion of the hood when the air is blown toward the operator. The constant flow of air out of the work area prevents contaminated room air from entering the work area.

b) **Vertical Flow Hoods** - air enters at the top of the unit and is blown downward in to the work area. Vertical flow hoods protect the technician from exposure to cytotoxic or hazardous drugs as well as maintain the sterility of the IV solution. For the preparation of hazardous drugs, a vertical flow hood must be used. Vertical Flow Hoods are also known as "Biological Safety Cabinets".

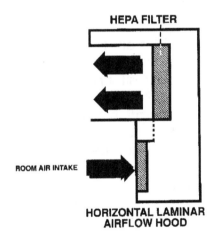

HEPA FILTER

ROOM AIR INTAKE

HORIZONTAL LAMINAR AIRFLOW HOOD

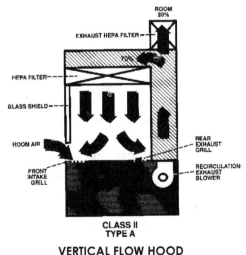

ROOM 30%

EXHAUST HEPA FILTER

70%

HEPA FILTER

GLASS SHIELD

ROOM AIR

REAR EXHAUST GRILL

FRONT INTAKE GRILL

RECIRCULATION/ EXHAUST BLOWER

CLASS II TYPE A

VERTICAL FLOW HOOD

The two types of vertical flow hoods are:
a) Class II Type A - exhausts 30% , HEPA filtered air back into room
b) Class II Type B - exhausts totally outside

NOTE: A critical principle of laminar flow use is that nothing must interrupt the flow of air between the HEPA filter and the sterile object. Objects placed between the HEPA filter and the sterile object may cause contamination of the sterile product. All manipulations of sterile products must be performed at least 6 inches within the hood. The technician should always work as far into the hood as possible without placing any portion of the body, with the exception of hands and forearms, inside the work environment. Laminar flow hoods should be left operating continuosly. If turned off, you must wait a minimum of 30 minutes before preparing sterile products once the hood is turned on. Before, after and at specified intervals during the use (see Policy and Procedure manual) of a laminar flow hood, all interior work surfaces should be cleaned with isopropyl alcohol or a suitable disinfecting agent. The work area should be cleaned from side to side, beginning at the back of the hood working your way to the front of the hood. Plexiglass sides of the hood may be damaged when cleaned with isopropyl alcohol and therefore other suitable disinfectants should be used. Laminar flow hoods must be inspected and certified by qualified personnel every 6 months or when damage is suspected.

ASEPTIC TECHNIQUE:
Although the laminar flow hood provides an aseptic environment, touch contamination has been shown to be the most frequent cause of contamination to IV admixtures. The following procedures for proper aseptic technique should be followed:
a) All personnel involved with preparation of sterile products should scrub their hands with a suitable antibacterial agent. Hands should be dried with disposable paper towels and not linen towels. A thorough scrubbing should be performed at least to elbow height including the finger nails and between fingers. This procedure should be repeated if contamination is suspected or when leaving and returning to the work area.
For Betadine or Hibiclens to be effective antimicrobial agents, contact with the skin must be for a period of at least several minutes.
b) Jewelry should not be worn on the hands or wrists when preparing sterile products since they may introduce contaminants into the work area.
c) Talking and coughing should be directed away from the laminar flow work area.
d) Only those objects needed for sterile product preparation should be brought into the laminar flow hood. Do not place labels, pens or medication orders onto the sterile work surface of the hood.
e) Trays should be washed on a regular weekly basis with a suitable agent to remove as much particulate contamination as possible.
f) Clean, particulate free garments should be worn when preparing sterile products. Gloves, masks, hair and shoe coverings may be required and will depend on individual institutional policies.
g) Avoid touching any portion of the sterile product. "Critical sites" of contamination are the needle shaft, syringe plunger and diaphragm of container.

SECTION 2C: TOTAL PARENTERAL NUTRITION (TPN)

The pharmacy technician must be aware of the factors that are involved in the destabilization of TPN solutions, as well as the chemical incompatibilities which may occur during the compounding process. This section will present the latest trends of current TPN technology, reviewing multiple approaches and theories commonly utilized in modern practice. The goal of a total nutrient admixture is to provide all necessary nutrients in a single container.

TPN CONTENTS: The components of an intravenous TPN admixture are:

1) **amino acids** - a source of building blocks for protein synthesis, amino acids provide the patient with 4 calories of energy per gram. Without sufficient amino acids for protein synthesis, the body is forced to break down muscle and other important proteins as a source of energy. Essential and nonessential amino acids refer to the body's ability to synthesize amino acids. Essential amino acids can not be synthesized by the body and must be provided nutritionally. Nonessential amino acids can be synthesized and are not a nutritional requirement. Aminosyn II, contains both essential and nonessential amino acids. Nephramine 5.4% and Aminosyn RF provide only essential amino acids intended for the use in patients with renal failure. Since these patients have difficulty excreting amino acids, these solutions are limited to essential amino acids only. Hepatamine is a specially formulated amino acid solution for the use in patients with compromised liver function.

2) **dextrose** - a poor source of energy, this carbohydrate provides the patient with only 3.4 calories per gram. Dextrose solutions are available commercially in several different concentrations, such as 5%, 10%, 20%, 50% and 70%. The most common percentage used in TPN is 50%, less in pediatric formulations and 20% for peripheral TPN.

3) **fats** - in the form of an emulsion, providing the largest amount of energy to the patient, 9 calories per gram. Due to the instability of early fat emulsions of the 70's and 80's, this component was generally piggybacked and not intimately mixed with the other ingredients of the TPN. With the advent of more stable fat emulsions and a clearer understanding of the factors causing this product to be unstable, TPN solutions are now commonly prepared in single 2-3 liter plastic bags as a complete 24 hour solution. A deficiency of one of the essentiall fatty acids, linoleic acid is associated with abnormal nail, hair and skin growth. Intralipid, Liposyn, Liposyn II and Soyacal are all available as 10% and 20% solutions and have been approved as stable fat emulsions by the FDA.

4) **electrolytes** - these include sodium, potassium, calcium, magnesium, chloride and phosphate.

5) **vitamins** - including the fat soluble vitamins (A,D,E) and the water soluble vitamins (B1, B2, B3, B5, B6, B12, C, folic acid and biotin).

6) **trace elements** - such as zinc, manganese, copper and chromium.

7) **others** - vitamin K, iron dextran, insulin, heparin and other medications.

FAT EMULSIONS: Intravenous fat emulsions are dispersions of immiscible liquids, "oil in water", which provide the patient with concentrated nutrients (9 calories per gram) and essential fatty acids (those fatty acids that the body cannot synthesize.

Two factors that contribute to the stability of these emulsions are:

1) **particle size** - As the particle size decreases, the physical stability of an emulsion increases. The majority of current lipid emulsions contain particle sizes ranging from 0.3 to 0.5 microns. This is why the use of a 0.22 micron in-line filter cannot be used with fat emulsions.

2) **pH** - Low pH results in emulsion destabilization by changing the coating of the lipid particles. These changes in the membrane surrounding the lipid particles results in a decrease of repulsive forces between particles which can lead to aggregation and coalescence. Coalescence and aggregation are similar terms referring to the formation of large lipid particles, that will either rise to the top (cream) or to be large enough to be visible as free oil floating on the surface of the emulsion.

There are 3 main ways that emulsions destabilize:

1) **creaming** - When intravenous fat emulsions are stored undisturbed for long periods of time, fat particles, which are lighter than water tend to rise toward the surface of the emulsion and appear as a chalky white cream layer. The solution at the bottom of the bottle may have a slightly bluish skimmed milk appearance. Slight shaking of the bottle will redisperse the lipid particles.

2) **aggregation** - When aggregation occurs, the repulsive forces between lipid particles have been replaced by attractive forces and they clump together. This process is also referred to as "flocculation" and may or may not be redispersible. This usually occurs when electrolytes or acidic solutions are added to fat emulsions. This process may or may not be visible to the naked eye.

3) **coalescence** - When droplets have been closely packed or aggregated, these droplets may combine to form larger droplets. This process involves loss or degradation of the membrane surrounding the droplet and a decrease in stability of the fat emulsion. This may or may not be visible to the naked eye and occurs most frequently when the emulsion has been frozen.

DEXTROSE: Solutions of dextrose are acidic. Since intravenous fat emulsions have no buffering capacity (the ability to resist change of pH upon the addition of acid or base) the addition of dextrose to the fat emulsion lowers the pH of the emulsion to that of the dextrose solution. This destabilizes the emulsion by changing the charge on the surface of the lipid particle, resulting in a loss of repulsive forces between particles and possible aggregation or flocculation.

AMINO ACIDS: Amino acid solutions are not disruptive to intravenous fat emulsions. In fact they have been found to exert a protective effect on the fat emulsion. Amino acids have a buffering capacity and help offset the negative effects of the low pH dextrose dilutions. It is thought that amino acids may form a mechanical barrier around the fat droplet thus preventing the destabilization of the fat emulsion.

ELECTROLYTES: Since the stability of the fat emulsion depends upon the repulsive forces of the negatively charged lipid particles, electrolytes, especially multivalent cations (positively charged ions) cancel out the negative charge of the lipid particles and cause unstable fat emulsions. They may be added to the amino acid solution or the dextrose solution before or after they are mixed with the fat emulsion. Iron dextran should never be added to lipid containing admixtures.

CALCIUM AND PHOSPHATE: Calcium and phosphate form insoluble precipitates under various conditions. Since TPN solutions are opaque, visual examination for precipitates is not possible. The factors that affect the solubility of calcium and phosphate are:
1) pH - is the most critical factor affecting insolubility, with higher pH's causing a greater degree of precipitate.
2) amino acid concentration - plays an important role in the formation of this precipitate, with increasing concentrations of amino acids causing less likelihood of formation of a precipitate.
3) temperature - precipitation is more likely at warmer temperatures. Therefore, TPN admixtures should be refrigerated immediately after compounding.

There are two approaches to overcoming this incompatibility:
1) Calcium should be added to the admixture last in order to provide maximum dilution of the phosphate before the calcium and phosphate come into contact with each other. If however, this process is reversed with the phosphate added to the solution containing calcium, the high localized concentration of phosphate may result in precipitation.
2) Instead of using calcium chloride as the source of calcium, calcium gluconate or calcium gluceptate should be used since these salts are less likely to cause this incompatibility. Even in this case, the calcium salts should be added to the admixture last.

VITAMINS AND TRACE ELEMENTS: Vitamins and trace elements should be added to the admixture just prior to the addition of the calcium. If possible, add both vitamins and trace elements into TPN admixtures immediately prior to administration. Total nutrient admixtures should be inspected carefully by the pharmacy technician following compounding and storage. The first and most obvious sign of an unstable admixture is creaming. The admixture will have a thick, chalky white cream layer on top of the container while the bottom of the container is frequently thin, watery and grayish in color. When the IV fat emulsion breaks, the color of the free oil may range from pale yellow to brown. Freshly prepared TPN admixtures, especially those containing multi-vitamins, are normally off-white or banana colored.

Orders for TPN admixtures should be written by the physician on specially prepared order sheets which express grams of protein, total calories, percent of calories from dextrose, percent of calories from fat, total volume, electrolytes, trace elements, multivitamins and any other additives "per 24 hours".

MEDICATIONS: Two medications commonly added to TPN admixtures are HEPARIN and INSULIN. Heparin is added to prevent the formation of blood clots (thrombosis) while insulin is added to help the patient utilize the large dextrose load. The physician monitors daily blood sugar and adjusts the amount of insulin added to the TPN. "The Guide to Parenteral Admixtures" is an excellent reference source for compatibility data when adding other medications.

COMPOUNDING:
The first principle is that of careful aseptic technique. A single container hung at the bedside for 12-24 hours provides an opportunity for significant microbacterial growth if contamination has occurred. Acceptable mixing techniques include:

1) The amino acids and dextrose are mixed together first. The fat emulsion is mixed with the amino acid solution and the additives are added last. It is also acceptable to incorporate the additive into the dextrose and amino acid solutions before combining them with the fat emulsion. In this instance, the calcium salts are added last to achieve maximal dilution prior to their addition.

2) The amino acids are added to the fat emulsion. To this admixture the dextrose is added. The additives are added last.

3) The dextrose, amino acids and fat emulsion are added simultaneously, gently swirling and mixing as the filling takes place. The additives are added last.

Automated compounding utilizes a pump to deliver exact amount of nutrient solutions from individual containers into a single final container. With this method there is little waste since reservoir bottles can be used for subsequent admixtures. Other advantages over the gravity method of compounding are accuracy and the ability to verify by computer printout each formula compounded, decrease in transfer time and total compounding time, as well as a decrease in the likelihood of unexpected incompatibilities. An example is Baxter's "AUTOMIX".

When a new TPN order is received in the pharmacy it must be reviewed and checked for accuracy and compatibility by a pharmacist before it is profiled and entered into the computer. The pharmacy technician should always review both the order and the label when receiving the TPN order from the pharmacist. The admixture should always be compounded according to the TPN order and not from the label.

CONTAINERS: At one time, TPN admixtures were mixed and administered from one liter glass bottles. This meant that three individual TPN containers were prepared daily for the patient and that admixtures were hung three times daily. One major disadvantage was that this increased the possibility of touch contamination of the admixture. Current practice is to combine the entire day's TPN, either with or without fat emulsion, in a single plastic bag which is hung at the bedside for 12-24 hours. Today, most bags which are designed for use with lipid-containing TPN admixtures are made from ethyl vinyl acetate (EVA), which contain no plasticizer at all.

ADMINISTRATION: Because TPN admixtures are extremely hypertonic, they are most commonly administered through a large central vein that leads directly to the heart. The subclavian vein located just beneath the clavicle (collarbone) is commonly used. Administration through a central line allows for the rapid dilution of this hypertonic admixture. Parenteral nutrition admixtures infused through a peripheral vein must be less concentrated (less hypertonic). A 10% dextrose concentration and 3-5 % amino acid concentration is regarded as the highest concentrations of dextrose and amino acids that should be administered via a peripheral vein. Even at these concentrations, the solution is irritating to the vein and may require changing the infusion site every couple of days.

There are two methods employed in starting and stopping parenteral nutrition admixtures:

1) The **rate** of administration is slowly increased over several days until a therapeutic volume is obtained. This allows for the pancreas to adjust to the increased dextrose load and the possibility of hyperglycemia.

2) The **concentration** of dextrose in the TPN admixture is slowly increased over several days until therapeutic concentrations of dextrose is achieved.

In either case, insulin may be added to the admixture to help the patient accommodate the extra dextrose load.

Likewise, in order to avoid hypoglycemia (low blood sugar), parenteral nutrition admixtures should never be discontinued abruptly. Patients should be tapered off TPN admixtures either by decreasing the administration rate over several days or by slowly decreasing the concentration of dextrose in the admixture.

TPN admixtures must be administered with an infusion pump to ensure a constant rate of infusion. If the fat emulsion is administered separately, a second pump is required and must be synchronized with the other solution. This is often a difficult, time consuming process. The use of several containers for a patient's daily means increased handling and increased probability of touch contamination.

After compounding,the TPN admixture must either be used immediately or stored in the refrigerator. The FDA has directed manufacturers to advise users to store TPN admixtures for no more than 24 hours in a refrigerator and to use them completely within 24 hours after removal from the refrigerator. With the advent of far more stable TPN admixtures currently in use, these limits may be exceeded. In no case should total nutrient admixtures remain at the bedside for longer than 24 hours.

SECTION 2D: SAFE HANDLING OF ANTINEOPLASTIC DRUGS

This section is an overview of the recommendations for the safe handling of parenteral antineoplastic and hazardous drugs as outlined by the U.S. Department of Health, Public Health Service and the National Institute of Health.

INTRODUCTION

The majority of antineoplastic drugs are toxic compounds. Many are known to cause carcinogenic, mutagenic, or teratogenic effects. On direct contact, some antineoplastic drugs may cause irritation to the skin, eyes, and mucous membranes, and ulceration and necrosis of tissue. The toxicity of parenteral antineoplastic drugs dictates that the exposure of medical personnel to these drugs should be minimized. At the same time, the requirement for maintenance of aseptic conditions during drug preparation must be satisfied. This section reviews routes through which exposure may occur and presents recommendations for the safe handling of parenteral antineoplastic drugs by pharmacists, pharmacy technicians and other personnel who are involved in the preparation and administration of these drugs to patients.

POTENTIAL ROUTES OF EXPOSURE

The potential routes of exposure during the preparation and administration of antineoplastic drugs are primarily through inhalation of the aerosolized drug and by direct skin contact. During the preparation of these drugs, a variety of manipulations are used which may result in aerosol generation, spraying, and splattering. Examples of these manipulations include:
- withdrawal of needles from drug vials;
- use of syringes and needles or filter straws for drug transfers;
- breaking open of ampules; and the expelling of air from a syringe when measuring the precise volume of a drug.

Good pharmaceutical practice calls for the use of aseptic techniques and a sterile environment when preparing parenteral drugs. Many pharmacies provide a sterile environment by using a horizontal laminar flow clean work bench. While this type of unit provides product protection, it exposes the operator, and other room occupants, to aerosols generated during drug preparation procedures. A Class II laminar flow (vertical) biological safety cabinet will provide both product and operator protection. This is accomplished by filtering incoming and exhaust air through high-efficiency particulate air (HEPA) filters. It should by noted that these filters are not effective for volatile materials, because the filters do not capture vapors and gases.

During administration, clearing air from a syringe or infusion line and leakage at tubing, syringe, or stopcock connections present obvious opportunities for accidental skin contact and aerosol generation. The practice of clipping used needles and syringes will also produce a considerable aerosol.

The disposal of antineoplastic drugs and trace contaminated materials (gloves, gowns, needles, syringes, vials, etc.), presents a possible source of exposure by these drugs to nurses, physicians, and pharmacists in addition to support and housekeeping personnel. Excrement from patients receiving certain antineoplastic drug therapy (e.g., high dose methotrexate) may contain high concentrations of the drug. Nursing personnel should be aware of this source of potential exposure to antineoplastic drugs and take appropriate precautions to avoid accidental contact. The potential risks to nurses, physicians, and pharmacists from repeated contact with parenteral antineoplastic drugs can be effectively controlled by a combination of specific containment equipment and certain work techniques. For the most part, the techniques are merely an extension of good work practices by medical personnel.

RECOMMENDED PRACTICES FOR PERSONNEL PREPARING PARENTERAL ANTINEOPLASTIC DRUGS

Professionally accepted standards concerning the aseptic preparation of parenteral products should be followed. Only properly trained personnel should handle antineoplastic drugs. Training sessions should be offered to new professionals as well as technical and housekeeping personnel who may come in contact with these agents. Safe handling should be the focus of such training.

1) All procedures involved in the preparation of parenteral antineoplastic drugs should be performed in a Class II laminar flow biological safety cabinet. Careful consideration should be given to selecting a cabinet size that will accommodate the preparation unit's work load.

2) Personnel should be familiar with the capabilities, limitations, and proper utilization of the biological safety cabinet selected. A Class II, Type A cabinet will provide product protection and prevent exposure of the operator to aerosols. The filtered exhaust from this type of cabinet is normally discharged into the room environment. Where possible, however, it is desirable to discharge the filtered exhaust air to the outdoors. This can be accomplished by installing an exhaust canopy over the Class II, Type A cabinet or by the use of a Class II, Type B biological safety cabinet which discharges exhaust air to the outdoors.

3) The safety cabinet work surface should be covered with plastic-backed a bsorbent paper. This will reduce the potential for dispersion of droplets and spills and facilitate clean-up. The paper should be changed after any overt spills and after each work shift. All materials used in the preparation of antineoplastic drugs must be disposed in specially marked biohazardous waste recepticals.

4) Personnel preparing the drugs should wear surgical gloves and a closed front surgical-type gown with knit cuffs. Gowns may be of washable or disposable variety. Contaminated gloves or outer garments should be removed and replaced. In case of skin contact with the drug, thoroughly wash the affected area with soap and water. Flush affected eye(s) with copious amounts of water for at least 15 minutes while holding the eyelid(s) open;then seek evaluation by a physician.

5) Vials containing reconstituted drugs should be vented to reduce internal pressure. This will help to reduce the possibility of spraying and spillage when a needle is withdrawn from the septum.

6) A sterile alcohol dampened cotton pledget should be carefully wrapped around the needle and vial top during withdrawal from the vial septum. Similarly, an alcohol dampened cotton pledget should be carefully placed at the needle or syringe tip when ejecting air bubbles from a filled syringe. This practice will control dripping and aerosol production which may occur during these procedures. AVOID SELF-INOCULATION. Take care when conducting any procedure that involves the use of needles.

7) The external surfaces of syringes and I.V. bottles should be wiped clean of any drug contamination.

8) When breaking the top off a glass ampule, wrap the ampule neck at the anticipated break point with a sterile alcohol dampened cotton pledget to contain the aerosol produced and also to protect fingers from being lacerated by the broken glass.

9) Syringes and I.V. bottles containing antineoplastic drugs should be properly identified and dated. When these items are delivered to a nursing ward, an additional label such as "Caution—Cancer Chemotherapy, Dispose of Properly" is recommended.

10) Wipe down the interior of the safety cabinet with 70% alcohol using a disposable towel after completing all drug preparation operations.

11) Contaminated needles and syringes should be disposed of intact, to prevent aerosol generation created by clipping needles. Place them in a leak-proof and puncture resistant container. This container, as well as contaminated bottles, vials, gloves, absorbent paper, disposable gowns, gauze, etc., should be placed in an appropriately labeled plastic bag-lined box, sealed and incinerated. Washable gowns may be laundered in a normal fashion.

12) Wash hands after removing gloves. Gloves are not a substitute for handwashing.

13) Remaining or left over antineoplastic drugs should be disposed of in accordance with Federal and State Requirements applicable to toxic chemical waste.

CHEMOSAFETY SPILL KITS
Chemosaftey Spill Kits are used to cleanup accidental spills of chemotherapeutic agents. These kits should contain the following items: waste disposal bags, respirator, saftey glasses, pair of latex gloves, heavy- duty utility gloves, absorbent toweling, gown, shoe covers, and sealable safelock bags.
A record should be kept describing the spill and should include the date, time, location, drug spilled and the amount spilled.

SECTION 3: FEDERAL PHARMACY LAW

A "pharmacy technician" is a certified, supportive personnel, who aids in delivering quality pharmacy services under the direct supervision of a licensed pharmacist. Even though some State Boards of Pharmacy have failed to recognize these important health care practitioners, vitally needed as the role of the pharmacist expands, others have shown acceptance through certification. <u>Mandatory education</u>, along with <u>certification</u>, set a standard of practice for this profession. The following section will provide an overview of technician functions and the legal considerations related to each of these tasks. The National Certification Exam tests the pharmacy technician on federal law only. One credit of continuing education in law is required for recertification (every 2 years).

FEDERAL REGULATIONS AND AGENCIES

1) FOOD, DRUG, and COSMETIC ACT (FDCA) - enacted in 1906, it prohibits the distribution or sale of "adulterated" or "misbranded" foods and drugs. Adulteration is defined as the presence of any decomposed substance, packaging under unsanitary conditions, or if the product's strength, quality, or purity is different from what is indicated on the label. Misbranding is defined as false or misleading labeling or when proper warnings and directions are absent. It is this legislation that oversees the marketing of all new drugs. A new drug application (NDA) must be filed to prove efficacy and safety before any drug is available commercially.

    a) DURHAM-HUMPHREY AMENDMENT (1951) - an amendment to the Food, Drug and Cosmetic Act (FDCA)separating drugs into 2 categories;
        1) *LEGEND DRUGS* - are drugs that bear the federal legend "Caution: Federal law prohibits dispensing without a prescription" and are restricted to sale and use under medical supervision.
        2) *NON-LEGEND DRUGS* - OTC or over - the - counter drugs that are not restricted to sale and use under medical supervision and do not bear the federal legend. The following information must appear on the label of a drug approved for OTC distribution:
            • product name
            • name and address of the manufacturer, distributor, repacker etc.
            • established name of all active ingredients and quantities of certain other ingredients whether active or not.
            • net contents of package
            • required cautions and warnings
            • name of any habit-forming drug in the product
            • adequate directions for use

b) KEFAUVER-HARRIS AMENDMENT (1962) - standardized labeling requirements for the manufacturer and dispenser to the patients. For labeling requirements, please see section #1. This amendment also regulates proper drug advertising and package inserts issued by the manufacturer. Manufacturers must register annually, be inspected at least once every 2 years and must report any drug reactions to the agency. Manufacturers must also follow standard investigational procedures for drug testing. Good Manufacturing Practices, GMP, were established with this legislation.

2) POISON PREVENTION PACKAGING ACT - this federal law was enacted to try and reduce accidental poisonings in children. All prescriptions filled by a pharmacy must be dispensed in child resistant containers. The exceptions to this legislation are the following;
   a) medications used for life-threatening medical emergencies, for example, nitroglycerin.
   b) written requests from prescriber or patients to dispense medications in nonchild resistant prescription containers.
   c) OTC medications clearly labeled "package not child resistant".
   d) patients who cannot open child resistant containers due to illness, for example, arthritic patients.

3) OMNIBUS BUDGET RECONCILIATION ACT (1990) - commonly referred to as OBRA, contains amendments to the Medicare/Medicaid programs funded by the federal government. The act requires the following:
   a) only drugs that are approved as safe and effective will be reimbursed.
   b) pharmacists must provide consulting services when dispensing medications.

4) CONTROLLED SUBSTANCE ACT (CSA) - Federal legislation (1970) regulating the use and distribution of drugs and other substances of abuse. It provides that controlled substances may only be distributed between persons who are registered with the Drug Enforcement Agency (DEA). The DEA is an agency of the U.S. Department of Justice and is responsible with the FDA for administering the provisions of the Controlled Substance Act.

The following activities requires registration with the DEA:
   a) manufacturing, distributing and dispensing of controlled substances
   b) conducting research and institutional activities with controlled substances
   c) conducting narcotic treatment programs
   d) importing or exporting of controlled substances
   e) compounding of a controlled substance

SCHEDULES
At the time the Controlled Substance Act of 1970 was enacted, Congress established five schedules of controlled substances based on:
   a) abuse potential (psychological and physical dependencies)
   b) accepted medical use

Substances in schedule I have the highest potential for abuse while substances in schedule V have a relatively low abuse potential. Commercial containers of controlled substances are required to be labeled with the letter "C" together with the Roman numeral of the schedule assigned to the substance. The federal transfer caution states "*Caution: Federal law prohibits the transfer of this drug to any person other than the patient for whom it was prescribed*".

SCHEDULE I:
- drugs or substances that have a high potential for abuse
- drugs or substances that have no currently accepted medical use
- drugs or substances that have a lack of accepted safety for use

Included within this schedule are certain opiate derivatives such as heroin and normorphine, some hallucinogens such as LSD, peyote and psilocybin. These substances may not be prescribed.

SCHEDULE II:
- drugs or substances that have a high potential for abuse
- drugs or substances that have accepted medical use
- drugs or substances that may lead to severe psychological or physical dependance

Included in this schedule is powdered opium, extracts of opium, cocaine, morphine, meperidine, codeine, Dolophine, dextroamphetamine, oxycodone, fentanyl, hydromorphone, pentobarbital, Marinol, Percodan, Percocet and Tylox. Schedule II substances are nonrefillable.

DEA FORM 222
To secure (purchase or transfer) a supply of schedule II substances, a registrant must complete DEA Form 222 triplicate order form. Triplicate order form booklets are issued by the DEA upon request. The order forms are serially numbered and include the registrant's name and address, DEA number, and the schedules the registrant is authorized to dispense. The order form is completed by the purchaser, who retains one copy and fowards two copies to the distributor, who in turn keeps one copy and fowards the last copy to the DEA. Any changes or erasures on DEA Form 222 voids the order form and will not be filled by the supplier. Only one supplier may be listed on one form. Only the person who signed the application for registration with the DEA is permitted to sign the order forms.

Schedule III:
- drugs or substances that have an abuse potential less than CI or CII
- drugs or substances that have an accepted medical use
- abuse that may lead to moderate - low physical dependence or high psychological dependence

DEA FORM 222

See Reverse of PURCHASER'S Copy for Instructions	No order form may be issued for Schedules I and II substances unless a completed application form has been received, (21 CFR 1305.04).		OMB APPROVAL NO. 1117-0010
TO: (Name of Supplier)		STREET ADDRESS	

CITY and STATE	DATE	TO BE FILLED IN BY SUPPLIER
		SUPPLIER'S DEA REGISTRATION No.

LINE No.	TO BE FILLED IN BY PURCHASER				Packages Shipped	Date Shipped
	No. of Packages	Size of Package	Name of Item	National Drug Code		
1						
2						
3						
4						
5						
6						
7						
8						
9						
10						

NO. OF LINES COMPLETED	SIGNATURE OF PURCHASER OR HIS ATTORNEY OR AGENT

Date Issued	DEA Registration No.	Name and Address of Registrant
Schedules	2, 2N, 3, 3N, 4, 5	
Registered as a PHARMACY	No. of this Order Form	

DEA Form (Jun. 1983) –222

U.S. OFFICIAL ORDER FORMS—SCHEDULES I & II
DRUG ENFORCEMENT ADMINISTRATION
SUPPLIER'S COPY 1

48

Schedule III (cont.)

Drugs in this class include Tylenol with Codeine I - IV, anabolic steroids, butisol, Deconamine DX, Didrex, Empirin with Codeine III - IV, Fiorinal, Hycodan, Hycomine, hydrocodone, Loracet, Loratab, Nucofed, Plegine, Synalgos DC, Tussend and Vicodin.

In 1990 anabolic steroids were added to this schedule. The definition of an anabolic steroid is any drug or hormonal substance, chemically and pharmacologically related to testosterone that promotes muscle growth.

Schedule IV:
- drugs or substances that have a low potential for abuse relative to substances in schedule III
- drugs or substances that have accepted medical use
- abuse may lead to limited physical or psychological dependence

Drugs in this class include the benzodiazepines such as alprazolam, clonazepam, diazepam, flurazepam, lorazepam, oxazepam and temazepam. Other CIV controlled substances include chloral hydrate, Cylert, Equagesic, Equanil, Luminal, phenobarbital, Sanorex and Wygesic.

Schedule V:
- drugs or substances that have a very low potential for abuse
- drugs or substances that have accepted medical use
- abuse may lead to limited physical or psychological dependence

The drugs in this schedule are generally antitussives and antidiarrheal medications. Examples of schedule V drugs are Tylenol/codeine Solution, Lomotil, Naldecon CX, Novahistine DH, Phenergan/codeine, Robitussin AC, Ryna C, Ryna CX, Actifed C, and Tussi-Organidin.

RECORD BOOK OF SALES OF NONPRESCRIPTION SCHEDULE V SUBSTANCES

In some states, certain controlled substances (primarily C-V substances) do not contain the federal caution and therefore are sold without a prescription. These preparations contain small amounts of controlled substances and the FDA feels that a prescription is not required. In some states, such as Colorado and N.Y. a prescription is required for CV substances.

To prevent abuse of these substances, the FDA has established certain guidelines for their sale and requires records of sale to be maintained.

The guidelines for sale of CV's include:
- the sale must be made by a licensed pharmacist
- the purchaser must be at least 18 years of age and must show suitable identification
- no more than 8 ounces or more than 48 dosage units of any substance containing opium in any 48 hour period may be dispensed to the purchaser. No more than 4 ounces or more than 24 dosage units of any other controlled substance in any 48 hour period may be dispensed to the purchaser.

The pharmacist must maintain a record of all such nonprescription sales in a bound book that contains the following regarding each sale:
- name and address of the purchaser
- name and quantity of the controlled substance
- date of purchase
- name or initials of the dispensing pharmacist

PRESCRIPTION FILING METHODS
Federal regulations provide for three methods of filing prescriptions.
1) Three separate prescription files:
- prescriptions for CII
- prescriptions for CIII-IV
- all other prescriptions

2) Two separate prescription files:
- prescriptions for CII - CV, provided that all CIII - CV contain a red "C" at least one inch high stamped in the lower right hand corner of the prescription
- all other prescriptions

3) Two separate prescription files:
- CII prescriptions only
- all other prescriptions, provided that all CIII - CV contain a red "C" at least one inch high stamped in the lower right hand corner of the prescription

The Controlled Substance Act requires that each pharmacy registrant make a complete and accurate inventory of all controlled substances every 2 years. The biennial inventory, which has been established as May 1, may be delayed for up to 6 months past the biennial date. The inventory must be maintained on site for at least 2 years.

VERIFYING CONTROLLED SUBSTANCE PRESCRIPTIONS
1) All prescription orders for controlled substances must be verified for authenticity by the pharmacist. Recognition of area prescribers, knowledge of the patient and careful review of the prescription contents should all be considered when establishing the validity of a prescription order.
2) Confirmation of the prescribers DEA # may aid in verifying the authenticity of a controlled substance prescription order. DEA #'s consist of 2 letters and 7 digits, with the second letter corresponding to the prescribers last name. If the first, third and fifth digits are added to two times the sum of the second, fourth and six digits the last digit of the total and DEA # will match.

example: DEA # = AH 1234563
a) 1 + 3 + 5 = 9
b) (2 + 4 + 6) x 2 = 24
c) 9 + 24 = 33
d) last digits of total must match last digit of DEA #

REFILLING OF CONTROLLED SUBSTANCES

a) Schedule II controlled substances may not be refilled. If the patient requires additional medication, a new written prescription must be issued by the prescriber. Oral prescriptions are permitted with the prescriber being responsible to provide a written "cover" prescription for each verbal order.

b) Schedules III and IV controlled substances may be refilled a maximum of 5 times within a 6 month period. Oral prescriptions are permitted for these Schedules.

c) Schedule V controlled substances must be recorded in a special "Schedule V Record Log" as previously indicated. For those states that require a prescription for Schedule V controlled substances, a maximum of 5 refills within a 6 month period is allowable. Oral prescriptions are also allowed.

LIMITATIONS OF PHARMACY TECHNICIAN DUTIES

Limitations of technician duties are set by individual state regulations. It is imperative that the technician know and understand the limitations dictated by their state law. According to federal regulations, the pharmacy technician may perform all functions of pharmacy practice under the assistance and direction of a licensed pharmacist except;

1) the pharmacy technician may not receive <u>oral prescriptions</u>
2) may not exercise <u>professional judgement</u> in any matter of pharmacy practice

SAFETY CONSIDERATIONS

Since the storage of drugs and chemicals occurs in the pharmacy workplace, attention must be paid to the safety of employees and consumers.
All pharmacies should:

1) post the number of their local poison control center within the dispensing area
2) have available a reference guide for toxicities related to the ingestion or topical exposure to medication or hazardous materials
3) provide Material Safety Data Sheets (M.S.D.S.) for any "hazardous materials" stored within the pharmacy. Material Safety Data Sheets are available from each manufacturer and describe in detail the procedures for ingestion or topical exposure and precautions for the products safe handling.

POISON LOG

Since the pharmacist is responsible for the sale of poisonous substances, a "poison log" must be kept for at least five years reflecting any sale of a poisonous material.

This log must include:

1) date of sale
2) name and address of purchaser
3) name and quantity of poison dispensed
4) reason for purchase
5) full name of dispenser

All poisonous substances must be labeled properly and must include:
1) the complete name of the particular poison
2) the word "POISON" boldly imprinted on its label
3) the place of business of the seller
4) proper directions for use

All pharmacies should be well stocked with one ounce bottles of "Syrup of Ipecac". Syrup of Ipecac should be used to induce vomiting (emesis) for noncaustic substances only. The dose is one tablespoonful (15ml) immediately after toxic ingestion and this dose may be repeated after 10-15 minutes if vomiting has not occurred. "Activated Charcoal" should be stocked by every pharmacy and is administered after toxic ingestion to adsorb and prevent absorption of the toxin and to serve as a marker for when the toxin was ingested. "Dilution" of a caustic substance with milk or any other suitable substance is the preferred method used to neutralize their caustic effects.

DRUG RECALLS
If a drug causes a severe adverse reaction or is improperly labeled by the manufacturer, the medical staff of the FDA determines the health hazard potential of the product and assigns a drug recall.
There are 3 classes of drug recalls:
A) **CLASS I** - where exposure to the product will cause a severe health hazard or death
B) **CLASS II** - where exposure to the product may cause a temporary or medically reversible adverse health hazard
C) **CLASS III** - where exposure to the product is not likely to cause an adverse health hazard

OCCUPATIONAL AND SAFETY ACT
The Occupational and Safety Act of 1970 ensures a safe and healthful workplace for all employees. Under this act falls the Occupational Safety and Health Administration (OSHA) which was created to:
1) develop mandatory job safety and health standards
2) maintain a reporting system for job related injuries and illness
3) decrease hazards in the workplace
4) conduct workplace inspections to ensure compliance with regulations

Several standards that relate to the practice of pharmacy are:
1) **Air Contaminants** - that may be inhaled when handling hazardous drugs or chemicals. OSHA has published its regulations in the reference "Guidelines for Cytotoxic (Antineoplastic) Drugs".
2) **Flammable and Combustible Liquids** - that must be stored in appropriate areas such as vaults or metal cabinets. Examples of flammable and combustible liquids are acetone, alcohol, ether-based solvents, etc. Proper quantity and placement of fire extinguishers must be available for immediate use in emergencies.
3) **Eye and Skin Protection** - for use when performing tasks that may produce flying objects such as glass, liquids or bodily fluids.

4) **Hazard Communication Standard (HCS)** - based on the concept that each employee has the need and right to know the hazards and identities of those chemicals or hazardous materials they may be exposed to in the workplace.

RULES FOR LEGAL JURISDICTION
To determine whether federal or state law has jurisdiction, the general rule is that the more stringent law should be followed.

PREPACKAGING OF MEDICATIONS:
The repacking of medications is common in most areas of pharmacy practice and usually involves the pharmacy technician. The technician must understand the stability and labeling requirements of prepackaging medications.
   1) **LABELING** - each repackaged drug must contain a label which includes the following information:
      a) generic name of the product
      b) strength
      c) dosage form
      d) manufacturer's name and lot number
      e) expiration date after repackaging (see below)

   2) **REPACKAGING LOG** - documentation required when prepacking functions are performed. All repackaged drugs must be carefully reviewed and documented by a licensed pharmacist before the drug is dispensed or put into stock. A log must be maintained which should include the following information:
      a) date of prepacking
      b) name of drug
      c) manufacturer
      d) manufacturer's expiration date and lot number
      e) quantity of drug repackaged
      f) licensed pharmacist's signature

   3) **EXPIRATION DATE OF REPACKAGED DRUGS** - federal law allows for the expiration date of a repacked medication not to exceed one year. This one year period must not exceed 50% of the remaining time between the date of repackaging and the expiration date on the original manufacturer's bulk container. Local state regulations may differ from federal law.

THE ORANGE BOOK
The Orange Book - Approved Drug Products with Therapeutic Equivalence Evaluations is a reference in which the FDA provides guidance to the pharmacist in generic drug product selection.

The Orange Book lists all sources of drug products grouped as "pharmaceutical equivalents". Pharmaceutical equivalents contain the same active ingredient in the same concentration, route of administration and dosage form. Drug products listed within equivalent categories are assigned a two-letter code.
      - drug products with the first letter code "A" are considered therapeutic equivalents
      - drug products with the "B" code indicate that the products have a documented therapeutic inequivalence

CENTER FOR DISEASE CONTROL (CDC)

The Center for Disease Control (CDC) is a federal agency which is a part of the Department of Health and Human Resources. It sets national standards for disease control and prevention. It provides statistics and information to health professionals on the treatment of common and rare diseases worldwide.
Its primary function is to issue regulations for infection control.

COMMON ABBREVIATIONS

AWP	Average Wholesale Price
CDC	Center for Disease Control
CSA	Controlled Substance Act
DEA	Drug Enforcement Agency
DME	Durable Medical Equipment
DUR	Drug Utilization Review
FDA	Food and Drug Administration
GMP	Good Manufacturing Practices
HCFA	Health Care Financing Administration
HHS	Department of Health and Human Services
IND	Investigational New Drug Application
MAC	Maximum Alllowable Cost
NDA	New Drug Application
NDC	National Drug Code
NIH	National Institutes of Health
OBRA	Omnibus Budget Reconciliation Act of 1990
OSHA	Occupational Safety and Health Administration
OTC	Over - the - Counter drug product
PPI	Patient Package Insert

SECTION 4: MEDICAL - PHARMACEUTICAL TERMINOLOGY AND ABBREVIATIONS

The pharmacy technician must be able to interpret medication orders in a variety of pharmaceutical settings. This includes community, institutional and home care settings. The student must memorize these abbreviations and symbols so that proper interpretation can be achieved.

MEDICALLY RELATED SYMBOLS

ABBREVIATION	INTERPRETATION
abd	abdominal
AIDS	acquired immunodeficiency syndrome
alb	albumin
alk	alkaline
ane	anesthesia
BM	bowel movement
BP	blood pressure
BS	blood sugar
CA	carcinoma
carb	carbohydrate
cath	catheter
CCU	coronary care unit
CHF	congestive heart failure
CNS	central nervous system
CVA	cerebro vascular accident
DX	diagnosis
ECG	electrocardiogram
EEG	electroencephalogram
EKG	electrocardiogram
FBS	fasting blood sugar
GI	gastrointestinal
HR	heart rate
ICU	intensive care unit
n&v	nausea and vomiting
NPO	nothing by mouth
post op	after surgery
post partum	after delivery
pre op	before surgery
STAT	now, at once
surg	surgery
TX	treatment
URI	upper respiratory infection
UTI	urinary tract infections

PHARMACEUTICALLY RELATED SYMBOLS

ABBREVIATION	INTERPRETATION
ADR	adverse drug reaction
amp	ampule
APAP	acetaminophen
APC	aspirin, phenacetin, codeine
ASAP	as soon as possible
AAWP	average, average wholesale price
AWP	average wholesale price
B+O	belladonna and opium
cmpd, cpd	compound
conc	concentration
DAW	dispense as written
DC	discontinue
DEA	Drug Enforcement Agency
DUR	drug utilization review
EtOH	ethyl alcohol, ethanol
HA	hyperalimentation
HC	hydrocortisone
HMO	health maintenance organization
INH	isoniazid
KVO	keep vein open
LAS	label as such
LCD	liquid carbonic detergent
legend	prescription drug
M.	mix
MAC	maximum allowable cost
MDI	metered-dose inhaler
mEq	milliequivalent
MOM	milk of magnesia
MS	morphine sulfate
MVI	multi-vitamin infusion
NF	National Formulary
NSAID	nonsteroidal anti-inflammatory drug
NTG	nitroglycerin
OJ	orange juice
OTC	over the counter
PCN	penicillin
ped.	pediatric
PPI	patient package insert
sat.	saturated
SSKI	saturated solution potassium iodide
T	temperature
TCN	tetracycline
TPN	total parenteral nutrition
USP	United States Pharmacopeia
vit	vitamin

COMMON ELEMENTAL SYMBOLS

SYMBOL	INTERPRETATION
Al	aluminum
Ag	silver
Au	gold
Ba	barium
Br	bromine
C	carbon
Ca	calcium
Cl	chlorine
Cr	chromium
Cu	copper
Fe	iron
H	hydrogen
I	iodine
K	potassium
Li	lithium
Mg	magnesium
Mn	manganese
N	nitrogen
Na	sodium
O	oxygen
P	phosphorous
Pb	lead
S	sulfur
Zn	zinc

COMMON CHEMICAL FORMULAS

FORMULA	INTERPRETATION
$AgNO_3$	silver nitrate
$Al(OH)_3$	aluminum hydroxide
Cl	chloride
CO_2	carbon dioxide
$FeSO_4$	ferrous sulfate
HCl	hydrochloric acid
H_2O_2	hydrogen peroxide
KCl	potassium chloride
KI	potassium iodide
$KMnO_4$	potassium permanganate
K_3PO_4	potassium phosphate
MgO	magnesium oxide
$MgSO_4$	magnesium sulfate
$NaCl$	sodium chloride
NaF	sodium fluoride
$NaHCO_3$	sodium bicarbonate
O_2	oxygen
PO_4	phosphate
SO_4	sulfate

DRUG INFORMATION SOURCES

1) American Drug Index - is an alphabetical listing of both single-entity and combination drugs cross referenced by generic, brand and chemical names. The monographs list the name of the product, the manufacturer, the use and the dosage, the dosage forms available and their size and strength.

2) Drug Topics-Red Book - is a guide to products and prices listing manufacturer, available sizes, strengths, wholesale and retail prices. This annual publication is alphabetized by both trade and generic names and contains a product identification chart as well as other reference tables.

3) Hansten's Drug Interactions - is a guide to drug-drug interactions and the effects of drugs on laboratory tests.

4) Facts and Comparisons - a monthly updated guide of pertinent data on actions, indications, warnings, interactions, contraindications, precautions, adverse reactions and dosage. The products are grouped by pharmacological use rather than being listed alphabetically or by manufacturer.

5) Handbook on Injectable Drugs - an ASHP publication on compatabilities, storage and reconstitution guidelines of all parenteral products.

6) Handbook of Non-Prescription Drugs - is an APhA handbook containing comprehensive information on OTC products. Products are grouped by use. It describes basic physiology of self-medicated disease states.

7) Merck Index - is an encyclopedia of chemical data related to drugs and other chemical substances. This alphabetical listing includes chemical names and formulas, chemical activity, medical activity and other names for products used worldwide.

8) Merck Manual - is an alphabetical arrangement of general disease categories and their treatments.

9) Physician's Desk Reference (PDR) - an annual publication providing essential information on major pharmaceutical products as prepared by the manufacturer.

10) Remington's Pharmaceutical Sciences - is the most comprehensive work in the area of the pharmaceutical sciences. It contains all information required for a variety of pharmacy settings.

11) U.S. Pharmacopeia - National Formulary (USP-NF) - is the combined official compendia of pharmacy practice. Contains standards for natural products as well as for synthetic drugs.

PATIENT PACKAGE INSERTS

Each manufacturer of prescription medications must provide a detailed package insert, either affixed to or inside the drug product. This information should include:
1) product description
    a) chemical properties b) physical properties
2) approved FDA indications for use
3) contraindications
4) warnings (extreme side effects)
5) precautions (less severe side effects)
    a) drug - disease interactions
    b) drug - drug interactions
    c) excretion within breast milk, pregnancy or birth defects

6) adverse reactions
    a) interference with lab data
    b) statistics involved with each side effect
7) dosage, administration and product information

Patient Package Inserts (PPI) are required to accompany certain medications each time they are dispensed. These medications include:
1) Metered-Dosed Inhalers
2) oral contraceptives
3) Accutane
4) estrogens
5) progesterones

STORAGE TEMPERATURES

Specific directions are given in the USP-NF with respect to the temperatures at which drugs and biologicals must be stored. Storage above or below these requirements may produce undesirable results. Therefore, the pharmacy technician must memorize and apply these standards when preparing and storing medications and biologicals.

1) **COLD** - any temperature not exceeding 8° C (46° F).
    a) Refrigerator - between 2° C and 8° C (36° F to 46° F).
    b) Freezer - between -20° C and -10° C (-4° F to 14° F).

2) **COOL** - any temperature between 8° C and 15° C (46° F to 59° F).
    a) any article specified for storage in a cool place may be stored at refrigerated temperatures unless specifically stated otherwise.

3) **ROOM TEMPERATURE** - the temperature prevailing in the work area.
    a) Controlled Room Temperature = thermostatically controlled between 15° C and 30° C (59° F to 86° F).

4) **WARM** - any temperature between 30° C and 40° C (86° F to 104° F).

5) **EXCESSIVE HEAT** - above 40° C (104° F).

6) **PROTECTION FROM FREEZING** - when freezing a product one or more of the following may result:
    a) breakage of container
    b) loss of strength or potency
    c) alteration of the dosage form

TEMPERATURE CONVERSIONS

The pharmacy technician may be required to convert from Centigrade to Fahrenheit (C to F) or from Fahrenheit to Centigrade (F to C). The following formula will allow the pharmacy technician to make this conversion.

$$9°(C) = 5°(F) - 160°$$

To solve for either C or F, apply basic algebraic principles of mathematics (see section on pharmacy mathematics).

TYPES OF WATERS

  1) **PURIFIED WATER USP** - water obtained by distillation, ion-exchange treatment, reverse osmosis or any other suitable process; contains no added substances. This is not intended for parenteral administration. Purified water must be used in the preparation and reconstitution of oral products.

  2) **WATER FOR INJECTION USP** - water purified by distillation or reverse osmosis. It contains no added substances. Water for Injection is not sterile and may not be used for the aseptic compounding of sterile products.

  3) **STERILE WATER FOR INJECTION USP** - water for injection that has been sterilized and suitably packaged. It contains no antimicrobial agent or other added substances. May be used for the preparation of parenteral solutions.

  4) **BACTERIOSTATIC WATER FOR INJECTION USP** - sterile water for injection containing one or more suitable antimicrobial agents.

  5) **STERILE WATER FOR IRRIGATION USP** - water for injection that has been sterilized and suitably packaged. It contains no antimicrobial agent or other added substance. This is commonly used to prepare irrigating solutions.

SECTION 5: DRUG CLASSIFICATION

The pharmacy technician must be able to categorize each drug into a major therapeutic classification and briefly be able to describe the therapeutic use of each drug. In addition, the pharmacy technician must know drug products by both their generic and trade names, be able to correlate proper dosage forms, strengths, routes, proper dosing intervals and storage requirements associated with each drug. The following section will list generic names followed by their corresponding trade names and a brief comment concerning the drug therapy.

ADRENOCORTICAL STEROIDS
The adrenal glands are located near the kidneys and contain two distinct parts: the adrenal cortex and the adrenal medulla. The adrenal cortex is the outermost part while the adrenal medulla is the middle portion. The adrenal cortex produces three major groups of hormones called steroids. They are:
(1) the mineralocorticosteroids, which regulate salt and water metabolism,
(2) the glucocorticoids, which have multiple actions, one of which is the reduction of the inflammatory response and (3) small amounts of sex hormones. Glucocorticoids dramatically reduce the manifestations of inflammation including the redness, swelling, heat and tenderness that are commonly present at the inflammation site. They are useful in the treatment of the symptoms of drug serum and transfusion reactions, bronchial asthma and allergic rhinitis (allergies). They also suppress the body's immune response and are used as adjuncts in chemotherapy. All oral inhalers must be shaken well before use and should contain the appropriate auxiliary label. Therapy with oral or parenteral steroids must never be stopped abruptly but must be withdrawn slowly.

ORAL AND PARENTERAL CORTICOSTEROIDS:

beclomethasone	QVAR	2 inhalations PO qid NO MORE THAN 10 INHALATIONS DAILY
beclomethasone	Beconase AQ	1 spray in each NOSTRIL bid-qid.
budesonide	Rhinocort	nasal spray "AQ" = AQUEOUS DOSAGE FORM
cortisone	Cortone	tabs, injection (susp). DOSAGES HIGHLY INDIVIDUALIZED
dexamethasone	Decadron	tabs, oral sol, elix, inj. "LA" = LONG ACTING 2 inhalations PO bid. DO NOT EXCEED 4 PER DAY
fluticasone	Flonase	nasal spray
hydrocortisone	Cortenema, Solu-Cortef, Cortef	tabs, inj, enema, susp,
methylprednisolone	Depo-Medrol, Solu-Medrol	tabs, inj

prednisolone	Orapred	tabs, syrup. retention
	Prelone	enema, inj, ophthalmin
		EXCRETED BY KIDNEY
prednisone	various	tabs, oral sol, oral conc, syr
	Deltasone	ORAL SOL.= 5mg/5ml
		CONCENTRATE= 5mg/ml
		METABOLIZED IN LIVER
triamcinolone	Aristocort, Kenalog	tabs, syr, inj, oral
	Nasacort	nasal aerosol
		intra-synovial, intralesional

TOPICAL CORTICOSTEROIDS:

amcinonide	Cyclocort	crm, lot, oint.
betamethasone	Diprolene	aerosol, crm, lot, oint.
clobetasol	Temovate	crm, lot, oint.
clocortolone	Cloderm	crm
desonide	Tridesilon	crm, oint, lotion
desoximethasone	Topicort	crm, gel, oint.
dexamethasone	Decaspray	aerosol
diflorasone	Psorcon, ApexiCon	crm, oint.
fluocinolone	Synalar	crm, oint, topical sol.
fluocinonide	Lidex	crm, gel, oint, topical sol.
hydrocortisone	various	1/2% and 1% = OTC
mometasone	Elocon	crm, oint, lotion
triamcinolone	Artistocort, Kenalog	aerosol, crm, lot, oint

Note: All topical preparations require "For External Use" auxiliary labels.
Infected areas should be cleansed prior to application.

ANALGESICS
a) NARCOTIC ANALGESICS

Used for the relief of pain (analgesia) by binding to opiate receptors at many sites within the CNS (brain and spinal cord), altering both the perception of and emotional response to pain. Receptors are thought of as specific binding sites on proteins or enzymes that elicit a response when a drug-receptor complex is formed. Auxiliary stickers warning of drowsiness and danger of concomitant use with alcohol must be affixed. The narcotic antagonist, naloxone, should always be available when using these drugs in case of accidental overdosing.

alfentanil	Alfenta	CII, injection only
butorphanol	Stadol	CII, injection only
	Stadol NS	nasal spray 10mg/ml
		COMMONLY USED
		PRE-OP AND POST-OP

codeine	codeine	CII, oral sol, tabs, inj, sol tabs. COMMONLY USED AS COUGH SUPPRESSANT
fentanyl	Sublimaze Duragesic Actiq Lozenges	CII, injection only. AVAILABLE AS TRANSDERMAL PATCHES 25, 50, 75 + 100mcg PER HOUR FOR 72 HOURS
hydromorphone	Dilaudid	CII, tabs, liq, inj, supp. HP IS HIGHLY CONC. FORM 10mg/ml
meperidine	Demerol	CII, tabs, syrup, inj. EFFECTIVE AS PARENTERAL
methadone	Dolophine	CII, tabs, inj, oral sol, dispersable tabs USED IN TX OF NARCOTIC WITHDRAWAL
morphine SO4	MS Contin	CII, tabs, oral sol, syrup, supp, ER tabs
nalbuphine	Nubain	injection only
oxycodone + ASA	Percodan Endodan	CII, tabs only. DEMI = CONTAINS 1/2 AMOUNT OF OXYCODONE
oxycodone + APAP	Percocet	CII, tabs, oral sol, supp.
oxymorphone	Opana	CII, tabs, ER
pentazocine	Talwin	CIV, tabs, inj.
naloxone + pentazocine	Talwin Nx	CIV, 50mg pentazocine + 500mg naloxone tabs only
sufentanil	Sufenta	CII, injection only

b) NON-NARCOTIC ANALGESICS AND ANTIPYRETICS

Used for the reduction of pain and fever, with some agents possessing antiinflammatory effects as well. These drugs produce analgesia either by inhibiting the synthesis of prostaglandin or inhibiting other substances that sensitize pain receptors to mechanical or chemical stimulation. It relieves fever by central action in the hypothalamic heat-regulating center of the brain. If the agent contains anti-inflammatory effects, it is thought to be due to inhibition of prostaglandin synthesis. The nonsteroidal anti-inflammatory drugs will be reviewed as a separate category and will be discussed in the next section.

acetaminophen	**"APAP"** various Tylenol	tabs, caps, supp, oral elix, syr, susp. CONTAINS NO ANTI-INFLAMMATORY EFFECT

acetylsalicylic acid	**"ASA"**	tabs, caps, EC, chew,
	various	supp, gum, powder.
	Aspirin	CONTAINS ALL THREE EFFECTS
diflunisal	Dolobid	tabs only.CONTAINS ALL THREE EFFECTS
phenazopyridine	Pyridium	tabs only - exerts
	AZO Standard	local anesthesia on urinary mucosa. COLORS URINE RED OR ORANGE

NONSTEROIDAL ANTI-INFLAMMATORY DRUGS

Produces anti-inflammatory, anti-pyretic (fever) and analgesic (pain) effects possibly through inhibition of prostaglandin synthesis. All these drugs should be taken with milk or food to minimize GI discomfort and therefore require a " Take With Milk or Food " auxiliary label. Are contraindicated in patients with peptic ulcer disease. To be used cautiously in patients taking the anticoagulant warfarin. Many products are enteric-coated and must not be crushed, broken or chewed.

celecoxib	Celebrex	caps, COX-2 Inhibitor
diclofenac	Cataflam	tabs, supp.
	Voltaren	
etodolac	Lodine(XL)	caps only. NOT FOR RHEUMATOID ARTHRITIS
fenoprofen	Nalfon	tabs, caps. MAY CAUSE DROWSINESS
flurbiprofen	Ansaid	tabs only. POSSIBLE CNS EFFECTS
ibuprofen	Advil	tabs, caplets, oral susp, OTC
	Motrin	RX NEEDED FOR 300mg
	Children's	OR GREATER
	Advil+Motrin	suspension, chew tabs, caplets
indomethacin	Indocin	caps, oral susp, inj.
ketoprofen	Orudis	tabs, (sustained-release), cap. ADMINISTERED ON EMPTY TOMACH
ketorolac	Toradol	tabs, inj.
meclofenamate	Meclomen	capsules
meloxicam	Mobic	tabs, suspension
nabumetone	Relafen	tabs only
naproxen	Naprosyn	tabs, oral susp, supp.
	Anaprox	DS=DOUBLE STRENGTH
	Aleve	OTC
oxaprozin	Daypro	tablets
piroxicam	Feldene	caps only. PHOTOSENSITIVITY COMMON
sulindac	Clinoril	tabs only
tolmetin	Tolectin	tabs, caps. DS = DOUBLE STRENGTH

ANTIANGINALS

Angina (pectoris) is a characteristic chest pain caused by coronary blood flow that is insufficient to meet oxygen demands to the heart muscle (myocardium). Angina is characterized by a sudden, severe substernal pain radiating down the left arm. Three categories of pharmacologic agents are used to treat angina pectoris: organic nitrates, calcium channel blockers and beta blockers.

a) ORGANIC NITRATES

This group of agents increase the blood flow in the cardiac muscle by relaxing coronary arteries

nitroglycerin	various Nitrostat	sublingual tabs + buccal tabs, caps = sustained-release, IV, topical oint, patches SL = DISP IN ORIGINAL GLASS ONLY. REPLACE Q3 MONTHS. IV = ALWAYS MIX IN GLASS CONTAINERS. USE NON-PVC TUBING. AVOID USE OF IV FILTERS
isosorbide dinitrate	Isordil Sorbitrate	tabs = sublingual, chewable + oral caps = immediate + sustained-release; SR + SA ARE BOTH SUSTAINED-RELEASE
isosorbide mononitrate	Imdur	24-hour oral tablet

b) CALCIUM CHANNEL BLOCKERS

The Ca++ channel blockers inhibit the entrance of calcium into cardiac muscle cells and thereby cause the blood vessels of the heart to vasodilate (open).

amlodipine	Norvasc	tabs only
diltiazem	Cardizem Dilacor	CD = dual-release caps; SR = extended injection at10mg/hr
felodipine	Plendil	oral only
nicardipine	Cardene	caps, sustained-release caps, inj.
nifedipine	Procardia Adalat	caps = immediate release tabs = sustained-release
nimodipine	Nimotop	oral only
nisoldipine	Sular	oral only,
nitrendipine	Bypress	oral only
verapamil	Calan Isoptin	tabs = immediate release inj. SR tabs = sustained-release

c) BETA BLOCKERS
The beta blocking agents suppress the activity of the heart by blocking beta 1 receptors. They also decrease the workload of the heart by causing a slight decrease in blood pressure.

- see section on antiarrhythmic agents for complete listing

ANTIARRHYTHMICS
The heart contains specialized cells that can automatically generate rhythmic impulses that cause the heart to beat. Dysfunction of the impulse generator (pacemaker) or conduction at any of a number of sites in the heart can cause the heart to slow down (bradycardia) or speed up (tachycardia). There are five classes of antiarrhythmic drugs, which are:

a) Class I = SODIUM CHANNEL BLOCKERS

disopyramide	Norpace	tabs = sustained-release; caps = immediate + sustained-release SUSPENSION COMPOUNDED FROM 100mg
dofetilide	Tikosyn	caps, MCG dosing CAPS. PROTECT FROM LIGHT
flecainide	Tambocor	tabs, injection MIX ONLY WITH D5W FOR IV INFUSION
ibutilide	Corvert	injection only
lidocaine	Xylocaine	injection only
mexilitine	Mexitil	caps, injection
moricizine	Ethmozine	tabs
procainamide	Pronestyl	tabs, SR tabs, caps, inj.
quinidine	various	tabs, sustained-release tabs, caps, inj. GI SIGNS OF TOXICITY
propafenone	Rythmol	tabs only

Note: The majority of these drugs should not be administered with cimetidine (Tagamet), for this is a significant drug interaction.

b) CLASS II = BETA-ADRENERGIC BLOCKERS

acebutolol	Sectral	caps
atenolol	Tenormin	tabs, inj.
betaxolol	Kerlone	tabs
bisoprolol	Zebeta	tabs
cartelol	Carteolol	tabs
esmolol	Brevibloc	injection only ULTRASHORT-ACTING AGENT; DO NOT ADM IV PUSH
labetolol	Trandate	tabs, inj.
metoprolol	Lopressor	tabs, inj.

nadolol	Corgard	tabs
pindolol	Visken	tabs
propranolol	Inderal	tabs (see antianginal section)
sotalol	Betapace	tabs
tomolol	Blocadren	tabs

c) CLASS III = POTASSIUM CHANNEL BLOCKERS

| amiodarone | Cordarone | tabs, inj. |
| bretylium | Bretylol | injection only |

d) CLASS IV = CALCIUM CHANNEL BLOCKERS

- see antianginal agents for complete listing

e) MISCELLANEOUS ANTIARRHYTHMIC AGENTS (USED IN TX OF CHF)

digoxin	Lanoxin	tabs, caps, elix, inj.
		PEDIATRIC INJ = 0.1mg/ml
digitoxin	Crystodigin	tabs only

ANTI-INFECTIVES

In general, the agents belonging to this category are used to either kill (bacteriocidal) or inhibit the growth of disease (bacteriostatic) causing (pathogenic)organisms. Since bactericidal agents are only effective against growing organisms, their effects are diminished when administered with bacteriostatic agents. Completing the full course of therapy is of the utmost importance and therefore the auxiliary label stating "Finish All Medications" or the specific duration of therapy should be placed on the prescription vial.

a) AMEBICIDES

chloroquine	Aralen	tabs, sc, IM, IV
eflornithine	Ornidyl	injection, ORPHAN DRUG
iodoquinol	Yodoxin	tabs only
		GIVE WITH FOOD.
		MAY CRUSH AND MIX
		IN APPLESAUCE OR
		CHOCOLATE SYRUP
furazolidone	Furoxone	oral liq, tabs
hydroxychloroquine	Plaquenil	tabs
mefloquine	Lariam	274mg tabs=250mg base
metronidazole	Flagyl	tabs, oral susp, inj.
		DO NOT USE WITH ALCOHOL
		= DISULFIRAM-LIKE REACTION
pentamidine	NebuPent	aerosol, inj.
	Pentam	FOR PCP OF AIDS-300mg
		AEROSOLIZED Q MONTH

b) AMINOGYLCOSIDES

This group exhibits its bacteriocidal effects by inhibiting protein synthesis in the pathogenic organism. They are nephrotoxic (kidney) and ototoxic (ear). Therefore, kidney function (BUN and creatinine clearance) must be monitored to determine the dosage and frequency of administration. Administration with any cephalosporin increases risk of nephrotoxicity. These agents are broad-spectrum antibiotics used mainly for the tough gram-negative organisms such as Pseudomonas, E. Coli, Proteus, Klebsiella and Enterobacter.

amikacin	Amikin	injection, ped inj. OK IF SOLUTION IS SLIGHTLY YELLOW
gentamicin	Garamycin	adult and ped inj, infusion MAY BE ADMINISTERED INTRATHECALLY. HEMODIALYSIS REMOVES 50% DRUG IN SERUM
kanamycin	Kantrex	caps, adult and pediatric inj. DILUTE 500mg in 200ml NS OR D5W
neomycin	various	tabs, oral sol. USED AS PRE-OP GUT STERILIZER
netilmicin	Netromycin	injection only
streptomycin		injection only USED IN COMBINATION WITH OTHER ANTITUBERCULAR AGENTS FOR TB.
tobramycin	Nebcin	adult and pediatric inj. nebulizer, premixed inf.

c) ANTIFUNGALS - SYSTEMIC

This group exhibits its antifungal activity by interfering with cell wall synthesis weakening the cell wall of the fungus or by interfering with protein synthesis (DNA or RNA). Many of these agents are hepatotoxic (liver) and liver function and enzymes must be monitored. It is not uncommon for therapy to last for several months.

amphoteracin B	AmBisome	inj.
fluconazole	Diflucan	tabs, inj. DO NOT MIX WITH ANY OTHER MEDICATIONS
flucytosine	Ancobon	caps - REFERED TO AS 5-FC
griseofulvin	Fulvicin, Grifulvin	tabs, caps, oral susp, micronized tabs. ABSORBED BEST WITH FATTY MEALS. MICRONIZED PROD HAS INC. ABSORPTION AND REQUIRES LOWER DOSES

itraconazole	Sporanox	caps inj, oral sol
ketoconazole	Nizoral	tabs, oral susp. NEEDS STOMACH ACIDITY TO BE DISSOLVED AND ABSORBED. NOT GIVEN WITH H2-BLOCKERS OR ANTACIDS.
metronidazole	Flagyl	tabs, inj
nystatin	Mycostatin, Nilstat	tabs, oral susp, loz, pwd, vaginal tablets
terbinafine	Lamisil	tabs

ANTIFUNGALS - TOPICAL

bacitracin	Various	ointment only CONTAINS NEOMYCIN 500 U/gm
cicloprox	Loprox Penlac	1% cream or lotion DON'T USE OCCLUSIVE DRESSING
clotrimazole	Lotrimin, Mycelex	1% loz, crm, top sol, vag crm + tabs ALL OTC PRODUCTS
econazole	Spectazole	1% crm
gentian violet		tampons=5mg, top sol 1% + 2% (OTC) WILL STAIN SKIN AND CLOTHING
ketoconazole	Nizoral	2% crm and shampoo.
miconazole	Micatin Desenex Zeasorb -AF	2% crm, lot, powd, spray, vag crm, vag tabs. All OTC.
nystatin	Mycostatin Nilstat	crm, oint, powd, vag tabs. REFRIGERATE VAGINAL TABS
oxiconazole	Oxistat	crm, lot.
terconazole	Terazol	3 = vag supp. 7 = vag crm.
tioconazole	Vagistat	6.5% vag oint.
tolnaftate	Tinactin	liq + powd aerosol, crm, gel, powd, top sol, pump spray, 1%, ALL OTC.
terbinafine	Lamisil	crm, spray
metronidazole	various	crm, emul, gel, lotion, vag gel

d) CEPHALOSPORINS

Usually bactericidal, these drugs inhibit cell wall synthesis of the disease causing organism. Structurally related to the penicillins and therefore used cautiously in patients who are sensitive or allergic to PCN. Must be properly dosed in patients with kidney impairment. For information on IV cephalosporins - see monographs in section 3.

cefaclor	Ceclor	caps, oral susp refrig, stable x14d MAY BE DOSED BID (Q12h)
cefadroxil	Duricef Ultracef	tabs, caps, oral susp = refrig x14d LONG 1/2 LIFE PERMITS QD TO BID DOSING
cefazolin	Ancef Kefzol	inj, infusion
cefoxitin	Mefoxin	injection
cefdinir	Omnicef	caps, susp.
cefditoran	Spectracef	tabs only
cefepime	Maxipime	inj. ADD-VANTAGE vial FOURTH-GENERATION CEPH.
ceftazidime	Fortaz	injection
ceftizoxime	Cefizox	injection
cefixime	Suprax	tabs, oral susp= stable x14d NO REFRIGERATION REQUIRED FOR SUSP
cefoperazone	Cefobid	infusion
cefotaxime	Claforan	injection
cefotetan	Cefotan	injection
cefpodoxime	Vantin	tabs, oral susp=refrig x 14d
cefprozil	Cefzil	tabs, oral susp= refrig x14d
ceftriaxone	Rocephin	injection
cefuroxime	Ceftin	tabs , susp, inj
cephalexin	Keflex	tabs, caps,oral susp=refrig x14d
cephradine	Anspor, Velosef	caps, oral susp=refrig x14d

e) ERYTHROMYCINS

This group is referred to as the macrolide antibiotics that bind to the 50S subunit of bacterial ribosomes, blocking protein synthesis. Can be bacteriocidal or bacteriostatic depending on the dose. Can be irritating to the stomach and therefore should be taken with food. Are commonly prescribed for patients allergic to penicillin.

ERYTHROMYCINS

azithromycin	Zithromax	tabs, inj, susp.
clarithromycin	Biaxin	film-coated tabs, XL TAKEN W/O REGARD TO MEALS
erythromycin	base	E-Mycin, Eryc, Eryc Sprinkle, PCE; tabs, caps, oral susp (must refrigerate)
erythromycin	Staticin, Emgel	topical for acne
erythromycin	Ilotycin	ophthalmic

erythromycin	estolate	Ilosone; caps, oral susp (must refrigerate)
erythromycin	ethyl succ	EES; (chew + granules) EryPed, Pediamycin
erythromycin	stearate	Erythrocin; tabs, oral susp (must refrigerate)
erythromycin	lactobionate	For IV or IM use only. DILUTE WITH STERILE WATER ONLY
erythromycin + sulfasoxizole	Pediazole	suspension only TAKE WITH FOOD OR MILK
telithromycon	Ketek	tabs,

f) PENICILLIN DERIVATIVES

Acts by preventing bacterial cell wall synthesis during active replication and is therefore bacteriocidal. They can be naturally or semisynthetically produced. The most common side effects are allergic type reactions such as rash, hives, or anaphylactic shock. All suspensions must be shaken well and refrigerated.

amoxicillin + clavulanate	Augmentin	chew tabs, tabs, oral susp. GI IRRITANT GIVE WITH FOOD. BROAD-SPECTRUM
amoxicillin	Various Amoxil	chew tabs, caps, oral susp. BROAD-SPECTRUM
ampicillin	Various	caps, oral susp, inj. BROAD-SPECTRUM
bacampicillin	Spectrobid	tabs only
carbenicillin	Geocillin	tabs only BROAD-SPECTRUM
cloxicillin	Tegopen	caps, oral susp. PENICILLINASE-RESISTANT
dicloxicillin	Dynapen, Dycil	caps, oral susp=62.5mg/5ml PENICILLINASE-RESISTANT
mezlocillin	Mezlin	inj.
nafcillin	Unipen, Nafcil	tabs,caps, oral susp, inj. PENICILLINASE-RESISTANT
oxacillin	Bactocil, Prostaphlin	caps, oral sol, inj. PENICILLINASE-RESISTANT
penicillin G,	Bicillin-LA	injection only benzathine REFRIGERATE IM ONLY NEVER ADMINISTERED IV
penicillin G, procaine	Wycillin	injection only procaine REFRIGERATE IM ONLY NEVER ADMINISTER IV
penicillin VK	Various	tabs, caps, oral susp.
piperacillin	Pipracil	inj.
ticarcillin	Ticar	injection only BROAD-SPECTRUM

g) TETRACYCLINES

Exerts bacteriostatic effect by binding to the 30s ribosomal subunit thus inhibiting protein synthesis. Antacids containing Al or Mg, calcium containing foods or iron containing products decrease the absorption by forming an insoluble complex. Expiration dates must be checked carefully because outdated tetracycline can cause kidney damage. Causes permanent tooth enamel discoloration and should not be taken during last half of pregnancy or by children under the age of eight. Causes photosensitivity and exaggerated sunburns. Use proper auxiliary labels to alert patient of these precautions. The tetracyclines are considered broad-spectrum antibiotics because of their wide range of antimicrobial activity.

doxycycline	Vibramycin	tabs, caps, oral susp, inj, syr. PROTECT FROM SUNLIGHT DURING INFUSION
minocycline	Minocin	tabs, caps, oral susp, inj.
tetracycline	various	tabs, caps, oral susp, inj.

h) ANTIVIRALS

Enters cell and becomes incorporated into viral DNA and there by inhibits multiplication. Viruses are intracellular parasites that lack both a cell wall and a cell membrane. Viral reproduction uses many of the hosts metabolic processes and few drugs are selective enough to prevent viral replication without injury to the host. Nevertheless, some drugs sufficiently discriminate between cellular and viral reactions to be effective and yet nontoxic. Viruses are not affected by antimicrobial agents.

abacavir	Ziagen	caps, tabs, susp, inj.
acyclovir	Zovirax	syr, caps, inj. NOW USED FOR CHICKEN POX
adefovir	Hepsera	tabs only
amantadine	Symmetrel	caps, syr, tabs. ONLY FOR INFLUENZA A VIRUS. USED IN TX OF PARKINSONISM
amprenavir	Agenerase	caps, oral sol.
atazanavir	Reyataz	caps only
cidofovir	Vistide	injection only
delavirdine	Rescriptor	tabs only
didanosine(ddI)	Videx	chew tabs, powd for oral sol - FOR HIV PATIENTS WHO NO LONGER RESPOND TO ZIDOVUDINE
efavirenz	Sustiva	caps, tabs.
emtricitabine	Emitriva	caps only
enfuvirtide	Fuzeon	injection only
famciclovir	Famvir	tabs only
fomivirsen	Vitravene	intravitreal injection
fosamprenavir	Lexiva	tabs only
foscarnet	Foscavir	inj.

ganciclovir	Cytovene	caps, inj. NOT IV OR IM
indinavir	Crixivan	caps only
lamivudine	Epivir-HBV	tabs, oral sol.
+zidovudine	Combivir	tabs only
lopinavir + ritonavir	Kaletra	caps, oral sol.
nelfinavir	Viracept	tabs, powder
nevirapine	Viramune	tabs, oral susp.
oseltamivir	Tamiflu	caps, oral sol.
ribavirin	Virazole	6gm in 100ml glass vial via inhalation.
rimantadine	Flumadine	tabs, syrup 50mg/5ml ASA OR APAP REDUCES SERUM LEVELS
ritonavir	Norvir	tabs, oral sol.
saquinavir	Inverase	caps only
stavudine (d4T)	Zerit	caps, oral sol.
tenofovir	Viread	tabs only
valacyclovir	Valtrex	caplets
vidarabine	Vira-A	inj concentrate 200mg/ml.
valganciclovir	Valcyte	tabs only
zalcitabine (ddc)	Hivid	tabs only (ddc) - MUST BE TAKEN WITH ZIDOVUDINE FOR ADVANCED HIV INFECTION.
zanamivir	Relenza	inhalation pwd
zidovudine (AZT)	Retrovir	caps, syr, inj, tabs. ADMINISTERED Q4h AROUND THE CLOCK

i) SULFONAMIDES

This class of antibiotics, commonly referred to as the "sulfa drugs", are normally bacteriostatic but may be bacteriocidal in large doses. They are usually administered orally since they are completely and rapidly absorbed from the GI tract. If oral administration is not possible, SC or IV sulfonamides may be administered. Because of the possibility of crystal formation in the kidney and urine (crystaluria) all patients must be aware of the need to drink plenty of water and can be cautioned to do so by affixing the appropriate auxiliary label. Should not be used together with ammonium chloride or vitamin C (ascorbic acid) since these agents acidify the urine and may cause crystaluria.

SMZ-TMP	Bactrim	80mg trimethoprim
	Septra	+400mg sulfamethoxizole
	Septra DS	160mg trimethoprim
	Bactrim DS	+800mg sulfamethoxizole tabs, oral susp, inj. "DS" OR "DF" = DOUBLE STRENGTH
sulfadiazine	Coptin	tabs only
triple sulfa	Sultrin	vaginal cream and vag tablets

sulfasoxazole	Gantrisin	oral tabs, susp. available as sterile ophthalmic solution and ointment
		pediatric liquid 500mg/5ml
sulfasoxazole + sulpafurazole	Novo-Soxazole	tabs

j) ANTIMALARIALS

Exact mechanism unknown but thought to bind and alter properties of DNA in susceptible parasites. If a person is traveling to endemic areas where malaria is common, treatment begins 2 weeks before entering area and continues eight weeks after leaving area. Visual disturbances such as blurred vision and difficulty focusing are common adverse reactions and should be monitored.

chloroquine	Aralen	tabs, syr, inj.
hydroxychloroquine	Plaquenil	tabs only.
mefloquine	Lariam	tabs only
pyrimethamine	Daraprim	tabs only.
quinine	various	tabs, caps.
		This drug also has skeletal muscle relaxation properties and is used to supress "leg cramping".

k) ANTITUBERCULARS

All these agents inhibit mycobacterial growth (the infective organism in TB) and are either bacteriostatic or bacteriocidal. These agents are rarely used alone but are used together, sometimes with as many as 5 drugs being taken at one time. Also the duration of therapy is usually long, ranging from 6 months to 2 years. These drugs are either used as primary, secondary, or tertiary agents.

cycloserine	Seromycin	capsules only. DO NOT USE WITH ALCOHOL. VIT B6 (PYRIDOXINE) SHOULD BE ADMINISTERED.
ethambutol	Myambutol	tablets only. NOT FOR CHILDREN UNDER 13 YEARS OLD
isoniazid	**"INH"** Nidrazid	tabs, oral sol, inj. VIT B6 SHOULD BE ADMINISTERED.
pyrazinamide	**"PZM"**	tablets only.
rifabutin	Mycobutin	capsules only

| rifampin | Rifadin, Rimactane | caps, inj. MAY TURN BODY SECRETIONS RED-ORANGE DO NOT USE WITH ALCOHOL |
| rifapentine | Priftin | tabs only |

ANTICHOLINERGIC AGENTS

The anticholinergic drugs bind to cholinergic receptors but do not elicit a response. When bound to the cholinergic receptor, the anticholinergic drug prevents acetylcholine from occupying that receptor site as well. Therefore, this group of drugs is also referred to as "cholinergic antagonists". The anticholinergic drugs are used clinically to decrease secretions in the GI system and block cholinergic stimulation in the heart thereby increasing heart rate and conduction, decrease bladder muscle spasms, decrease respiratory secretions and increase pupil size for ophthamalogical examinations. They are also used in the treatment of Parkinson's disease.

atropine	Atropisol	an agent in numerous preps ANTIDOTE = PHYSOSTIGMINE
dicyclomine	Bentyl	tabs, caps, syr, inj. - NOT SC or IV
belladonna	Belladonna Tinct USP	27-33mg alkaloid/ 100ml in 67% alcohol
benztropine	Cogentin	tabs, inj. USED FOR SIDE EFFECTS OF ANTIPSYCHOTICS
glycopyrrolate	Robinul (Forte)	tabs, inj, FORTE = 2mg
hyoscyamine	Levsin	tabs, caps, elix, oral sol, DROPS
scopolamine	Transderm-Scop	TRANSDERMAL PATCH PLACED BEHIND EAR FOR MOTION SICKNESS.

Agents used to increase pupil size (mydriatics) during eye examinations are discussed below.

atropine	IsoptoAtropine	ophth oint (OO)+sol (OS)
cyclopentolate	Cyclogel	ophth sol
epinephrine	Epifrin, Glaucon	ophth sol
homatropine	IsoptoHomatropine	ophth sol
scopolamine	IsoptoHyoscine	ophth sol

NEUROMUSCULAR BLOCKING AGENTS

This group of anticholinergic compounds block the transmission of nerve impulses to skeletal muscle. This group is used extensively for preoperative (pre-op) skeletal muscle relaxation. Since breathing involves the diaphragm, paralysis of the diaphragm with these agents will cause apnea ("a"= without,"pnea"= breathing).

atracurium	Tracrium	injection only
cisatracurium	Nimbex	injection only
doxacurium	Nuromax	injection only
mivacurium	Mivacron	inj, infusion
pancuronium	various	injection only - STORE IN REFRIGERATOR. DO NOT STORE IN PLASTIC SYRINGES OR CONTAINERS
rocuronium	Zemuron	injection only
succinylcholine	Anectine	injection only
	Quelicin	STORE INJECTABLE FORM IN
	Sucostrin	REFRIGERATOR

ANTICOAGULANTS

The drugs in this pharmacolgical class stop or slow the coagulation process (clotting) of blood. When blood clots form, they travel to various organs causing such disease states as stroke (brain), myocardial infarction (heart), pulmonary embolism (lung) or thrombophlebitis (vein). Close monitoring of patients taking these drugs is essential or the patient may "bleed to death".

dalteparin	Fragmin	injection only
enoxaprin	Lovenox	S.C. injection only
heparin	various	injection only PROTAMINE SO4 = ANTIDOTE
warfarin	Coumadin	tabs, inj. VITAMIN K = ANTIDOTE

ANTICONVULSANTS

Epilepsy (seizure disorder) is widespread in the general population (0.6%) affecting approximately 1.5 million people in the United States alone. It is a CNS disorder characterized by an abnormal and excessive discharge of signals in specific areas of the brain. It is not uncommon for seizures to be controlled with more than one anticonvulsant agent. More than 8 types of seizures are catagorized in current medical literature. Three agents, valproic acid, carbamazepine and lamotrigine are currently used in practice as MOOD STABILIZERS. These agents must never be withdrawn abruptly.

carbamazepine	Tegretol	tabs, oral susp. MILD MOOD STABILIZER
clonazepam	Klonopin	tabs, drops, inj. BENZODIAZEPINES MAY CAUSE DROWZINESS
diazepam	Valium	tabs, inj., FOR ACUTE USE ONLY.
divalproex	Depakote	E.C. + E.R. tabs, sprinkle CURRENT INDICATION AS MOOD STABILIZER

gabapentin	Neurontin	caps, oral sol
lamotrigine	Lamictal	tabs only
levetiracetam	Keppra	tabs, oral sol
oxcarbazepine	Trileptal	tabs, oral susp
phenobarbital	various	tabs, caps, oral sol, elix, inj. DO NOT MIX WITH ACIDIC DRUGS. MAY CAUSE DROWSINESS
phenytoin	Dilantin	tabs, oral susp, caps, inj. KAPSEALS = EXTENDED-RELEASE DO NOT MIX WITH D5W or IV INFUSION WITH IN-LINE FILTER. SHAKE WELL
primidone	Mysoline	tabs, oral susp.
valproic acid	Depakene	syr.

ANTIDIABETIC AGENTS

The pancreas produces the polypeptide hormone insulin which helps maintain homeostasis (balance) of blood glucose levels. A relative or absolute lack of insulin can cause serious hyperglycemia which is referred to as "diabetes mellitus". There are two types of diabetics: (1) insulin dependent diabetics (Type I), who do not produce any insulin and require daily injections and (2) non-insulin dependent diabetics (Type II), who produce very little insulin. Non-insulin diabetics receive oral hypoglycemic agents which cause increased production of insulin from the pancreas. Insulin is commercially available from various sources (pork, beef, human) having a varied onset and duration of action (rapid, intermediate and long acting). Storage in the refrigerator is NOT required but will prolong its shelf-life, and therefore an auxiliary label "Store in Refrigerator" should be affixed to all insulin preparations. All patients on oral hypoglycemic therapy should avoid any intake of alcohol and should be warned of such with the appropriate auxiliary label.

acarbose	Precose	tabs only
chlorpropamide	Diabinese	tabs only
glimepiride	Amaryl	tabs only
glipizide	Glucatrol	tabs only
+ metformin	Metaglip	tabs only
glucagon	E-Kit/Diag Kit	injection only
glyburide	Diabeta	tabs only
+ metformin	Glucovance	tabs only
insulin	various	injection only REGULAR, 70/30 LISPRO, LENTE UlTRALENTE, rDNA ONLY REGULAR IN IV INFUSIONS
metformin	Glucophage	tabs only
miglitol	Glyset	tabs only
nateglinide	Starlix	tabs only

pioglitazone	Actos	tabs only
repaglinide	Prandin	tabs only
rosiglitazone	Avandia	tabs only
+ metformin	Avandamet	tabs only
tolazamide	Tolinase	tabs only
tolbutamide	Orinase	tabs only

ANTIDIARRHEALS

These agents are used to stop diarrhea. No agent should be administered for longer than 48 hours without relief of diarrhea. For persistant diarrhea, a physician must be notified.

bismuth subsalicylate	Pepto-Bismol	chew tabs, oral susp. CONTAINS LARGE AMOUNTS OF SALICYLATES
diphenoxylate/atropine	Lomotil	tabs, liq. SCHEDULE V
kaolin/pectin	Kaopectate, Donnagel	oral susp
loperamide	Imodium	liq, caplets, OTC
opium tincture	Paregoric	oral sol camphorated SCHEDULE III

ANTIEMETIC AGENTS

This group of drugs is used to control nausea and vomiting (n+v) associated with pregnancy, chemotherapy, gastroenteritis, anesthesia and surgery. Their actions are thought to be due to inhibition of the chemoreceptor trigger zones and/or the vomiting center (VC) of the brain.

aprepitant	Emend	caps only
dimenhydrinate	Dramamine	tabs, elix,inj, syr.
dolasetron	Anzemet	tabs, inj.
dronabinol(delta-9-THC)	Marinol	caps only - MARIJUANA DERIV
meclizine	Antivert	tabs, caps.
	Bonine	ANTIHISTAMINE - MAY CAUSE DROWSINESS
metoclopramide	Reglan	tabs, syr, inj. INVESTIGATIONAL FOR N+V
ondansetron	Zofran	tabs, inj, oral sol
palonosetron	Aloxi	injection only
prochlorperazine	Compazine	tabs, syr, SR caps, supp, inj. ANTIHISTAMINE - MAY CAUSE DROWSINESS
promethazine	Phenergan	oral, IM, IV rectal suppository

trimethobenzamide	Tigan	caps, supp. inj. MAY CAUSE DROWSINESS. MAY CONTRIBUTE TO REYE'S SYNDROME. NOT FOR CHILDREN

ANTINEOPLASTIC AGENTS

Also referred to as anticancer drugs or chemotherapy, this group of drugs either kills or suppresses the active disease. It is estimated that 25% of the population of the United States will face a cancer diagnosis during their lifetime. An overall 5 year remission is considered a cure for a specific cancer. Since most pharmacy technicians are not involved with the preparation of these drugs, this topic will be limited to generic/trade and and common abbreviations.

GENERIC NAME	ABBREVIATION	TRADE NAME
altretamine	HMM	Hexalen
anastrozole	------	Arimidex
azathioprine	——	Imuran
bicalutamide	------	Casodex
bleomycin	——	Blenoxane
busulfan	——	Myleran
capecitabine	——	Xeloda
carboplatin	——	Paraplatin
carmustine	BCNU	BiCNu
chlorambucil	——	Leukeran
cisplatin	CDDP	Platinol
cyclophosphamide	CPM,CTX,CFT	Cytoxan
cytarabine	Ara-C	Cystosar-U
dacarbazine	DTIC	DTIC-Dome
dactinomycin	——	Cosmegen
diethylstilbestrol	DES	Stilphostrol
doxorubicin	——	Adriamycin
epirubicin	——	Ellence
estramustine	——	Emcyt
etoposide	VP16	Vepesid
exemestane	——	Aromasin
fludarabine	——	Fludara
fluorouracil	5FU	Efudex
fluoxymesterone	——	Halotestin
fulvestrant	——	Faslodex
gemcitabine	——	Gemzar
goserelin	——	Zoladex
hydroxyurea	——	Hydrea
idarubicin	PFS	Idamycin
ifosfamide	——	Ifex
letrozole	——	Femara
leuprolide	——	Lupron
lomustine	CCNU	CeeNu
mechlorethamine	nitrogen mustard	Mustargen
megestrol	——	Megace
melphalan	L-PAM	Alkeran
mercaptopurine	6-MP	Purinethol
methotrexate	MTX	Trexall
mithramycin	——	Mithracin
mitomycin	——	Mutamycin
mitotane	------	Lysodren
mitoxantrone	——	Novantrone

nilutamide	____	Anadron
oxaliplatin	EU	Eloxatin
paclitaxel	------	Taxol
pegaspargase	PEG-L	Oncaspar
procarbazine	____	Matulane
tamoxifen	____	Nolvadex
testosterone	____	Teslac
thiotepa	TESPA	Thioplex
toremifene	____	Fareston
vinblastine	VLP	Velban
vincristine	VCR	Oncovin

ANTIHYPERTENSIVE AGENTS

Hypertension is defined as a sustained diastolic blood pressure (pressure during relaxation of the heart) greater than 90 mm Hg accompanied by an elevated systolic blood pressure (pressure during the contraction of the heart) greater than 140 mm Hg. Hypertension is an extremely common disorder affecting approximately 15% of the population of the United States (60 million people). Although the majority of these individuals have no symptoms, chronic hypertension can lead to congestive heart failure (CHF), myocardial infarction, renal damage and stroke. The agents in this group will be categorized by their mechanism of action.

a) DIURETICS

These agents increase urinary excretion of sodium and water, thereby lowering blood pressure. Many diuretics also cause the excretion of potassium and therefore require concomitant potassium supplementation.

acetazolamide	Diamox	tabs, ext-release caps, inj. USED FOR GLAUCOMA
amiloride	Midamor	tabs only
bumetanide	Bumex	tabs, inj.
ethacrynic acid	Edecrin	tabs, inj.
furosemide	Lasix	tabs, oral sol, inj. ORAL SOLUTION STORED IN REFRIGERATOR
hydrochlorthiazide	HCTZ	tabs, caps, oral sol.
indapamide	Lozol	tabs only
mannitol	Osmitrol	inj. 5, 10, 15, 20, 25% OSMOTIC
metazolone	Zaroxolyn	tabs only
spironolactone	Aldactone	tabs only POTASSIUM SPARING DIURETIC. COMMONLY USED IN CHF
torsemide	Demadex	tabs, inj.
triamterene	Dyrenium	tabs. POTASSIUM-SPARING DIURETIC NO K+ SUPPLEMENT REQ.

b) BETA BLOCKING AGENTS

Beta blocking agents reduce blood pressure primarily by decreasing cardiac output and slowing heart rate. They also produce their antihypertensive action by causing relaxation of the blood vessels. This group of drugs are never abruptly discontinued and should be withdrawn over a two week period.

- see antiarrhythmic agents for complete listing

c) ACE INHIBITORS

Angiotensin-converting enzyme is the enzyme responsible for converting angiotensin I to angiotensin II. Angiotensin II is the most potent vasoconstrictor (agent that causes the blood vessels to narrow or constrict) in the body causing an increase in blood pressure. By inhibiting this enzyme, the body produces less angiotensin II, thereby lowering blood pressure.

benazepril	Lotensin	tabs only FATTY MEALS INHIBIT ABSORPTION
captopril	Capoten	tabs only, TID, AC DOSING
enalapril	Vasotec	tabs, inj.
fosinopril	Monopril	tabs only
lisinopril	Prinivil, Zestril	tabs only
perindopril	Aceon	tabs only
quinapril	Accupril	tabs only
ramipril	Altace	caps only
tandolapril	Mavik	tabs only

d) CALCIUM CHANNEL BLOCKERS

- See section on antianginal agents for complete listing

e) OTHER AGENTS:

clonidine	Catapres	tabs. TRANSDERMAL PATCHES (TTS) PATCH PROVIDES 7 DAYS OF CONTINUOUS THERAPY
diazoxide	Hyperstat	injection only PROTECT IV SOLUTIONS FROM LIGHT.
guanabenz	Wytensin	tabs only. INVESTIGATIONAL FOR OPIATE WITHDRAWAL
hydralazine	Apresoline	tabs, inj. USED FOR ECLAMPSIA OF PREGNANCY
methyldopa	Aldomet	tabs, oral susp,,inj.

minoxidil	Loniten	tabs, topical sol. CAUSES HAIR GROWTH
nitroprusside	Nipride	injection only WRAP IV INJECTION WITH FOIL
prazosin	Minipres	capsules only USED TO TREAT RAYNAUD'S DISEASE

ANTIPARKINSONIAN AGENTS

Parkinson's disease is a progressive disorder of muscle movement, characterized by tremors, muscular rigidity, slowness in carrying out voluntary movements and postural and gait abnormalities. It is a disorder caused by the death of a group of brain cells that use dopamine as its chemical transmitter.

amantadine	Symmetrel	tabs, syr. CONTAINS ANTIVIRAL PROPERTIES
benztropine	Cogentin	tabs, inj. USED FOR SIDE EFFECTS OF ANTIPSYCHOTICS
bromocriptine	Parlodel	tabs, caps. SHOULD BE TAKEN WITH MEALS
carbidopa+levodopa	Sinemet	tabs, CR = sust.-release
+entacapone	Stalevo	tabs only
levodopa	Larodopa	CARBIDOPA REDUCES AMOUNT OF LEVODOPA NEEDED
levodopa + carbidopa		tabs,
pergolide	Permax	tabs only
pramipexole	Mirapex	tabs only
procyclidine	Kemadrin	tabs only
ropinirole	Requip	tabs only
selegiline	Eldepryl	tabs, caps
tolcapone	Tasmar	tabs only
trihexylphenidyl	Artane	tabs, elix.

THYROID HORMONES

Thyroid hormones (thyroxine, T4) affect protein synthesis, glucose and carbohydrate metabolism, lipid metabolism, energy storage, body temperature and many other physiological processes. When the thyroid does not secrete enough hormone (hypothyroid), replacement therapy is required.

levothyroxine	Synthroid Levoxyl	tabs, inj. PREPARE IV DOSAGE IMMEDIATELY BEFORE ADM.
liothyronine	Cytomel	tabs only
thyroid dessicated	Armour Thyroid	tabs, caps.

82

ANTIULCER DRUGS

GI ulcers occur due to loss of tissue lining those parts of the digestive tract exposed to gastric acids. The drugs used to treat ulcers work by either reducing the secretion of gastic acids (H2 antagonists) or by coating the lining of the stomach and small intestines to protect it from the adverse effects of stomach acid.

cimetidine	Tagamet	tabs, oral liq, inj. DO NOT GIVE WITH ANTACIDS
famotidine	Pepcid	tabs, powder for oral susp, inj. ORAL SUSP = NO REFRIGERATION NEEDED. DISCARD AFTER 30 DAYS
esomeprazole	Nexium	ER caps
lansoprazole	Prevacid	ER caps NOT FOR MAINTENANCE THERAPY
misoprostol	Cytotec	tabs only
nizatidine	Axid	capsules only MAY OPEN CAPSULES AND MIX WITH JUICES. AVOID MIXING WITH TOMATO-BASED JUICES
pantoprazole	Protonix	tabs, inj.
omeprazole	Prilosec	capsules only delayed-release SWALLOW WHOLE. DO NOT OPEN OR CRUSH
rabeprazole	ACIPHEX	ER tabs
ranitidine	Zantac	tabs, syr, inj, infusion INCOMPATABLE WITH ALUMINUM. AVOID ALUMINUM-BASED NEEDLES
sucralfate	Carafate	tabs. NOT ADM WITH ANTACIDS

BRONCHODILATORS

This group of drugs affects the respiratory system either by acting directly on the bronchial airways or affecting the central nervous system (CNS) areas that control respiration. Those drugs acting on the respiratory tree most often relax bronchial smooth muscle and are commonly used to treat asthma.

albuterol	Proventil Ventolin	tabs, syr, sol for nebulizer AEROSOL INHALER
aminophylline	various	tabs, CR tabs, oral sol, inj.

epinephrine	Adrenalin	aerosol inhaler, inj. INJECTABLES CONTAIN VARIOUS CONCENTRATIONS; DO NOT MIX WITH ALKALINE SOLUTIONS
ipratropium	Atrovent	inhaler, sol for nebulizer
isoproterenol	Isuprel	inhaler, neb sol,inj. SL tabs
levalbuterol	Xopenex	inhalant sol.
metaproterenol	Alupent	tabs, oral sol, inhaler, neb sol
pirbuterol	Maxair	inhaler only
salmeterol	Serevent	inhalant aerosol NOT FOR ACUTE THERAPY
tertbutaline	Brethine	tabs, inj.
theophylline	various	tabs, chew tabs, ext-release tabs, caps, ext-release caps, elix, oral sol, inj.

DRUGS USED IN SHOCK

When the effective volume of blood in the circulatory system is sufficiently decreased, blood pressure will drop. This may be due to actual hemorrhage, rapid loss of blood or to an increase in the size of the circulatory bed. The drugs used in treating shock exert a stimulatory effect on the heart causing it to beat faster (chrontropic) and have a more forceful contraction (inotropic). They also cause the blood vessels to vasoconstrict thereby increasing blood pressure.

dobutamine	Dobutrex	injection only DO NOT MIX WITH SODIUM BICARBONATE see monograph in section 3
dopamine	Intropin	injection only DO NOT MIX WITH OTHER DRUGS

LAXATIVES

Laxatives and cathartics are used to promote defecation in patients with constipation. They are often used prior to certain medical procedures to empty the colon. There are five categories of laxatives which are classified as follows:

a) IRRITANTS

These agents irritate the smooth muscle of the intestine and cause increased peristalsis (increase muscular activity).

bisacodyl	Dulcolax	tabs, enema, supp. TABS ARE ENTERIC-COATED DO NOT CRUSH OR CHEW

cascara	various	tabs, fluid extract MAY DISCOLOR URINE
castor oil	various	oral liquid, emulsion

b) SALINE CATHARTICS
Produces an osmotic effect in the small intestine by drawing water into the intestine.

magnesium citrate	Citroma	oral solution CHILL TO MAKE MORE PALATABLE
sodium phosphates	Phospo-soda	liq, enema USED AS PHOSPHATE REPLACEMENT. USED TO TREAT HYPERCALCEMIA

c) BULK-FORMING
These agents absorb water and expand to increase bulk and moisten contents of stool. The increased bulk promotes peristalsis and bowel movement.

calcium polycarbophil	FiberCon Mitrolan	tabs, chew tabs. TAKE WITH FULL GLASS OF WATER
methylcellulose	Citrucel	powder, tabs.
psyllium	Metamucil	chew tabs, effervescent powder and granules, wafers, powder MIX WITH AT LEAST 8 OUNCES OF LIQUID

d) FECAL SOFTENERS
These are surface-active agents that reduce surface tension of the liquid contents of the bowel causing the incorporation of additional liquid in the stool.

docusate Na	Colace	caps, liq, syr enema conc. COMMONLY REFERRED TO AS DSS

e) LUBRICANTS
Agents that lubricate the bowel thereby preventing water from being absorbed out of the bowel.

mineral oil	Kondremul	oral liq, emulsion, DO NOT ADMINISTER TOGETHER WITH FAT SOLUBLE VITAMINS (A,D,E,K) OR COLACE

PSYCHOTHERAPEUTIC AGENTS

a) ANTIANXIETY AGENTS
These agents reduce anxiety by depressing the CNS at the limbic and subcortical levels of the brain. These drugs are also used as sedatives (ability to calm) and hypnotics (causing sleep) depending on the dose administered. The auxiliary labels stating "Do Not Drink Alcoholic Beverages" as well as "May Cause Drowsiness" should be affixed to the prescription container.

alprazolam	Xanax	tabs, oral sol.
buspirone	BuSpar	tabs only
diazepam	Valium	tabs, caps (extended-release), inj.
hydroxyzine	Atarax Vistaril	tabs, caps, oral susp, syr, inj.
lorazepam	Ativan	tabs, inj.
midazolam	Versed	injection only
oxazepam	Serax	tabs, caps.

b) ANTIDEPRESSANTS
Depression is an affective disorder characterized by a change in mood. The symptoms of depression are intense feelings of sadness, hopelessness, despair and the inability to experience pleasure in usual activities. All antidepressants work by changing the concentrations of chemical transmitters in the brain.
Effects of these agents usually takes 2 weeks or longer.

amitriptyline	Elavil	tabs, inj.
bupropion	Wellbutrin	tabs, SMOKING CESSATION
citalopram	Celexa	tabs, sol.
desipramine	Norpramine	tabs, caps.
doxepin	Sinequan	caps, oral concentrate
escitalopram	Lexapro	tabs, oral sol.
fluoxetine	Prozac	caps, oral sol.
imipramine	Tofranil	tabs, caps, inj.
mirtazapine	Remeron	tabs, disintegrating tabs
maprotiline	Ludiomel	tabs only
nortriptyline	Pamelor	tabs, caps, oral sol.
paroxetine	Paxil	tabs, susp. - FOR OCD
sertraline	Zoloft	tabs, caps, oral concentrate
trazadone	Desyrel	tabs only
venlafaxine	Effexor	tabs, caps

c) ANTIPSYCHOTICS
Also referred to as neuroleptics or major tranquilizers. These agents are used to treat psychosis and schizophrenia. Behaviors typically include delusions, hallucinations and agitation. Extrapyramidal side effects (EPS) and tardive dyskinesia (TD) are common. When stopping therapy these drugs must be tapered slowly.

86

aripiprazole	Abilify	tabs - MONITOR FBS
chlorpromazine	Thorazine	tabs, oral conc. caps sustained-release
clozapine	Clozaril	tabs only - WBC's weekly/biwkly
fluphenazine	Prolixin	tabs, oral conc, elix, inj, oral conc.
haloperidol	Haldol	tabs, inj, oral conc.
loxapine	Loxitane	tabs, caps, oral conc, inj.
olanzapine	Zyprexa	tabs, inj, disint. tabs
perphenazine	Trilifon	tabs, syr, oral conc, inj.
pimozide	Orap	tabs only
quetiapine	Seroquel	tabs only
risperidone	Risperdal	tabs, sol, disint. tabs
thioridazine	Mellaril	tabs, oral susp CONCENTRATE = 30mg/ml
thiothixene	Navane	caps, oral conc, inj.
trifluoperazine	Stelazine	tabs, oral conc, inj.
ziprasidone	Geodon	caps, inj.

VITAMINS

VITAMIN	**NAME**	**USE**
vitamin A	retinol	retinal function, bone growth
vitamin B1	thiamine	carbohydrate metabolism
vitamin B2	riboflavin	tissue respiration
vitamin B3	niacin	lipid metabolism
vitamin B6	pyridoxine	amino acid metabolism
vitamin B9	folic acid	red blood cell formation
vitamin B12	cyanocobalamin	red blood cell formation
vitamin C	ascorbic acid	collagen formation, tissue repair
vitamin D2	ergocalciferol	absorption + utilization of Ca^{++} and $PO4$
viitamin D3	cholecalciferol	absorption + utilization of Ca^{++} and $PO4$
vitamin E	---------	antioxidant
vitamin K1	phytonadione	blood clotting
vitamin K3	menadione	blood clotting

NOTE: The fat-soluble vitamins are A, D, E, and K while the water-soluble vitamins are vitamins B and C.

TRACE ELEMENTS

chromium
copper
iodine
mangenese
selenium
zinc

SECTION 6: PHARMACEUTICAL MATHEMATICS

This section takes a step-by-step approach to pharmaceutical mathematics and will provide the pharmacy technician with all methods necessary in dealing with pharmacy math. Remember that common mistakes in simple mathematics can lead to dosing errors and possible harm to the patient.

(I) Basic Mathematics:

1) Fractions

A fraction is a portion of a whole number. The top number is called the "numerator", while the lower number is called the "denominator".

$\underline{1}$ = numerator
2 = denominator

A fraction whose numerator and denominator are multiplied or divided by the same number does not change the value of the fraction. If the numerator and denominator are multiplied by the same number, the fraction is said to be "enlarged" yet still maintains it's same value. If the numerator and denominator are divided by the same number, the fraction is said to be "reduced" yet still retains it's same value.

$\dfrac{2 \times 2}{4 \times 2} = \dfrac{4}{8}$ Enlarging

$\dfrac{2 \div 2}{4 \quad 2} = \dfrac{1}{2}$ Reducing

Reducing Fractions: Find the largest number that can be divided evenly into both the numerator and denominator. Patience is required to reduce large fractions since finding the largest number may be difficult. Therefore, you may have to reduce several times.

Reduce $\dfrac{189}{216}$

First $\dfrac{189 \div 3}{216 \div 3} = \dfrac{63}{72}$

then $\dfrac{63 \div 9}{72 \div 9} = \dfrac{7}{8}$

Types of Fractions:

a) ***proper fraction*** - the numerator is smaller than the denominator.

example: $\dfrac{2}{5}$

b) ***improper fraction*** - the numerator is larger than the denominator.

example: $\dfrac{5}{2}$

Note: To change an improper fraction into a mixed number, just divide the denominator into the numerator and reduce the remaining fraction.

example: $\dfrac{5}{2} = 5 \div 2 = 2\dfrac{1}{2}$

c) ***mixed fraction*** - contains a whole number and a fraction.

example: $2\dfrac{3}{5}$

Note: Prior to performing any mathematical function, the mixed fraction must be converted to an improper fraction. This is accomplished by multiplying the whole number by the denominator and then adding the numerator. This number becomes the numerator and is placed over the stated denominator.

example: $2\dfrac{3}{5} = \dfrac{2 \times 5 + 3}{5} = \dfrac{13}{5}$

d) ***complex fraction*** = fraction contained in both the numerator and denominator.

example: $\dfrac{\frac{2}{5}}{\frac{1}{3}}$ equals $\dfrac{2}{5} \div \dfrac{1}{3}$

Note: This type of complex fraction may be solved by inverting the fraction in the denominator and multiplying.

example: $\dfrac{\frac{2}{5}}{\frac{1}{3}}$ equals $\dfrac{2}{5} \times \dfrac{3}{1} = \dfrac{6}{5}$

Functions involving fractions:

a) ***Adding or subtracting fractions***

• Find the lowest common denominator. If the lowest common denominator cannot be found, multiply the numerator and denominator of the first fraction by the denominator of the second fraction, and the numerator and denominator of the second fraction by the denominator of the first fraction.

- Add or subtract the numerators only. The denominator remains the same.

- Reduce to lowest terms.

example: $\frac{2}{3} + \frac{1}{4} = \frac{2 \times 4}{3 \times 4} + \frac{1 \times 3}{4 \times 3} = \frac{8}{12} + \frac{3}{12} = \frac{11}{12}$

$\frac{1}{2} - \frac{1}{3} = \frac{1 \times 3}{2 \times 3} - \frac{1 \times 2}{3 \times 2} = \frac{3 - 2}{6} = \frac{1}{6}$

b) *Multiplying fractions*

- Multiply the numerators.

- Multiply the denominators.

- Reduce to lowest terms.

example: $\frac{2}{3} \times \frac{1}{4} = \frac{2 \times 1}{3 \times 4} = \frac{2}{12} = \frac{2 \div 2}{12 \div 2} = \frac{1}{6}$

c) *Dividing fractions*

- Invert (turn upside down) the fraction following the division sign.

- Change division sign to multiplication.

- Multiply numerators and denominators.

- Reduce to lowest terms.

example: $\frac{2}{3} \div \frac{1}{4} = \frac{2}{3} \times \frac{4}{1} = \frac{2 \times 4}{3 \times 1} = \frac{8}{3} = 2\frac{2}{3}$

Note: When multiplying or dividing by a whole number, change the whole number into a fraction by placing the whole number over one and thereby making it into a fraction. Then just follow the rules outlined above.

example: $4 = \frac{4}{1}$

Changing fractions to decimals:
This can be accomplished by dividing the numerator by the denominator. In division, the number being divided is called the "dividend"; the number that does the dividing is called the "divisor"; the answer is referred to as the "quotient". Remember 1/4 can be read as 1 ÷ 4.

example:
$$1/4 = 4\overline{)1.00} = 0.25$$

$$\begin{array}{r} 0.25 \\ \hline 1.00 \\ \underline{8} \\ 20 \\ 20 \end{array}$$

Changing decimals to fractions:

This can be accomplished by placing the decimal over 100 and then reducing the fraction.

example: $0.25 = \dfrac{25}{100} = \dfrac{25 \div 25}{100 \div 25} = \dfrac{1}{4}$

2) Decimals

The majority of medication orders are written in the metric system. Most pharmacy calculations involving drug dosing utilize the metric system. It is essential that the pharmacy technician understand and master calculations involving decimals.

Multiplying decimals:

• Multiply the numbers as though the decimal is not present.

• Count the number of spaces to the right of the decimals in the numbers multiplied.

• Move the decimal point in the answer one place to the left for each number of spaces counted to the right of the decimal.

• Remember, a whole number contains an imaginary decimal to the right of the whole number (i.e. 2 is the same as 2.0).

example: 4.267 3 numbers are to the right of decimal
              x 2.4 1 number to the right of the decimal
              17068
            + 85340
            102408. move decimal 4 places to the left

10.2408   = correct answer

Dividing decimals

Remember, the number being divided is called the dividend; the number that does the dividing is called the divisor, and the answer is called the quotient.

$$\begin{array}{r} 22. \text{ -- quotient} \\ \text{divisor--}15\overline{)330.} \text{ -- dividend} \\ \underline{30} \\ 30 \\ \underline{30} \\ 0 \end{array}$$

Clearing the divisor of a decimal

Before dividing one decimal by another, the divisor must be cleared of decimal points.

- Move the decimal in the divisor to the far right counting the number of places the decimal has moved.

- Move the decimal in the dividend the same number of places to the right.

- Bring up the decimal point to its proper repositioned place.

$$\text{example: } \frac{0.004}{0.2} = 0.2\overline{)0.004} = 2\overline{)00.04}^{\,0.02}$$

Addition of Decimals

Unlike the multiplication of numbers containing decimals, when adding numbers with decimals, the decimal must be lined up properly in a straight line before addition can occur.

- Rewrite the problem lining up the decimal points.

- Add the same as with whole numbers.

example: 2.2 + 0.04 + 5.34

$$\begin{array}{r} 2.2 \\ 0.04 \\ + \underline{5.34} \\ 7.58 = \text{answer} \end{array}$$

Subtraction of decimals

Follow the rules of addition using subtraction.

example: 46.72 - 0.4

$$\begin{array}{r} 46.72 \\ - \underline{0.4} \\ 46.32 = \text{answer} \end{array}$$

Decimals and multiples of ten

When a number containing a decimal is either multiplied or divided by 10, 100, 1000 or any multiple of 10, then only the decimal moves to the right or to the left.

a) **Division** - when dividing, you make the number smaller. Therefore, move the decimal to the "left" as many places as there are zeros in the divisor.

example: 645.32 ÷ 10   = 64.532
        645.32 ÷ 100   = 6.4532
        645.32 ÷ 1000 = 0.64532

b) **Multiplication** - when multiplying, you make the number larger. Therefore, move the decimal to the "right" as many places as there are zeros in the multiplier.

example: 7.8637 x 10   =   78.637
         7.8637 x 100   =   786.37
         7.8637 x 1000   = 7863.7

3) **Roman Numerals:**
Roman Numerals can be included in 3 possible areas within the prescription order:

a) to designate a strength or quantity of a drug.
i.e. codeine SO4 ii gr.

b) to specify the number of doses.
i.e. tabs V

c) to indicate an amount of a drug in the directions.
i.e. ii gtts ou bid

VALUES OF ROMAN NUMERALS

ROMAN NUMERAL	VALUE
$\overline{ss}$	1/2
I or i	1
V or v	5
X or x	10
L or l	50
C or c	100
D or d	500
M or m	1000

Rules for the use of Roman Numerals:

1) If a smaller number preceeds a larger number, then the number is subtracted.
i.e. CM = 900, IV = 4, XL = 40

2) If an equal or smaller number appears after a larger number, then the number is added.
i.e. XV = 15, LX = 60, XXVII = 27

(II) **WEIGHTS AND MEASURES**

METRIC SYSTEM:

The metric system is a decimal system based on tens that has three basic units of measurements:

MEASURE OF WEIGHT

MEASURE	ABBREVIATION	EQUIVALENT
gram	gm or g	1000 mg
milligram	mg or mgm	1/1000 gm
		0.001 gm
		1000 mcg
microgram	mcg or ug	1/1,000.000 gm
		0.001 mg
		1/1000 mg
kilogram	kg	1000 gm

MEASURE OF VOLUME

MEASURE	ABBREVIATION	EQUIVALENT
liter	L or l	1000 mL
milliliter	ml	1/1000 L
		0.001 L

MEASURE OF LENGTH

MEASURE	ABBREVIATION	EQUIVALENT
meter	m or M	1000 mm
		100 cm
centimeter	cm	1/100 m
		10 mm
millimeter	mm	1/1000 m

Conversions within the metric system

1) Changing grams to milligrams:
   - Move the decimal point 3 places to the RIGHT.

   - **HINT:** Think of the alphabet. When moving from the letter **G** to **M** in the alphabet you are moving to the RIGHT. Therefore, when converting from **G**rams to **M**illigrams, move the decimal 3 places to the RIGHT.

   - When moving a decimal where no number exists, just add zeros.

   example: Convert 1.5 gm to mg
   A B C D E F **G** H I J K L **M** N O P
   $\longrightarrow$

   1.5 gm = 1.500 = 1500 mg
   $\longrightarrow$

2) Changing milligrams to grams:
- Move the decimal point 3 places to the LEFT.

- **HINT:** Think of the alphabet. When moving from the letter **M** to **G** in the alphabet you are moving to the LEFT. Therefore, when converting from **M**illigrams to **G**rams, move the decimal 3 places to the LEFT.

example: Convert 200 mg to gm.

A B C D E F **G** H I J K L **M** N O P
←

200 mg = 200. = 0.200 gm
←

3) Changing milligrams to micrograms:
- Move the decimal 3 places to the RIGHT.
- **HINT**: Think of the alphabet. The last letter in MILL**I** is an **I** while the last letter in MICR**O** is an **O**. When moving from I to O in the alphabet you are moving to the RIGHT. Therefore, move the decimal 3 places to the RIGHT.

example: Convert 2 mg to mcg.

A B C D E F G H **I** J K L M N **O** P
→

2 mg = 2.000 = 2000 mcg
→

4) Changing micrograms to milligrams:
- Move the decimal 3 places to the LEFT.

- **HINT:** In the alphabet, when moving from the letter **O** to **I** you are moving to the LEFT. Therefore, move the decimal 3 places to the LEFT.

example: Convert 200 mcg to mg.

A B C D E F G H **I** J K L M N **O** P
←

200 mcg = 200. = 0.2mg
←

APOTHECARY SYSTEM:

The apothecary system of measurement was brought to the United States from England in colonial times. Some physicians still order medications this way and certain pharmacy practices use the apothecary system. The basic solid measure in this system is the grain (gr), while the basic fluid measure is the minum.

APOTHECARY MEASURES OF WEIGHT

MEASURE	EQUIVALENT
20 grains	1 scruple
8 drams	1 ounce
12 ounces	1 pound

APOTHECARY MEASURES OF LIQUID

MEASURE	EQUIVALENT
60 minums (m)	1 fluid dram (fl dr)
8 fluid drams	1 fluid ounce (fl oz)
	480 minums
16 fluid ounces	1 pint (pt)
2 pints	1 quart (qt)
4 quarts	1 gallon
	128 fluid ounces

Note: The minum should not be confused with the drop since they are not equivalent. In addition to this, notice that in the apothecary system the unit is written first, followed by the quantity.

example: gr x = 10 grains   or   iss = 1+1/2 drams

HOUSEHOLD MEASURES

All directions for patient use must be written in understandable terminology in order for the medication to be administered properly. The pharmacy technician must be able to convert from metric and apothecary systems to the common household system.

HOUSEHOLD MEASURES

MEASURE	EQUIVALENT
1 teaspoonful (tsp)	5 milliliters (ml)
1 tablespoonful (tbs)	15 ml
1 fluid ounce (fl oz)	30 ml
1 shotglass	60 ml
1 pint (pt)	473 ml
1 gallon (gal)	3785 ml
2.2 pounds (lbs)	1 kilogram (kg)
1 lb	454 gm

CONVERSIONS AMONG METRIC, APOTHECARY AND HOUSEHOLD SYSTEMS:

COMMON CONVERSIONS AMONG SYSTEMS

1 grain (gr)	65 mg
1 gram (gm)	15.4 gr
1 kilogram (kg)	2.2 lbs
1 meter (m)	39.4 inch
1 inch	2.54 cm
1 ounce apoth.	31 gm

(III) SOLVING FOR X:

When solving for an unknown quantity (which we will call X), only one of four basic operations will be required to solve for the unknown. The question you ask yourself is "what is being performed to X in this equation?" Whatever function is being performed to X, you perform the inverse or opposite function and X will be solved. Remember, if 2 quantities are equal to each other then the same mathematical function may be performed to both sides of the equation without changing it.

Let's review solving for an unknown.

   a) ***Multiplication of X*** = If X is multiplied by a number, to solve for X, just divide by the same number as X is being multiplied.

   example: 5X = 30

In the above equation, X is being multiplied by 5. Therefore, to solve for X, divide both sides of the equation by 5.

$$\frac{5X}{5} = \frac{30}{5}$$

Remember, any number divided by itself is equal to 1.

X = 6

   b) ***Division of X*** = If X is being divided by a number, to solve for X, just multiply both sides of the equation by that number.

   example: $\frac{X}{6} = 7$

In the above equation, X is being divided by 6. Therefore, to solve for X, just multiply both sides of the equation by 6.

$$\frac{(6)X}{6} = 7(6)$$

X = 42

c) *Addition to X* = If a number is added to X, then to solve for X, just subtract that number from both sides of the equation.

example: X + 4 = 7

In the above equation, 4 is being added to X. To solve for X, subtract 4 from both sides of the equation.

$$X + 4 = 7$$
$$\underline{- 4 \quad -4}$$
$$\mathbf{X = 3}$$

d) *Subtraction from X* = If a number is being subtracted from X, then to solve for X, just add that number to both sides of the equation.

example: X - 8 = 7

In the above equation, 8 is being subtracted from X. Therefore, to solve for X, add 8 to each side of the equation.

$$X - 8 = 7$$
$$\underline{+ 8 \quad +8}$$
$$\mathbf{X = 15}$$

RULE: If more than one function is being performed to X in one equation, first add or subtract, then multiply or divide.

example: $\dfrac{3X}{4} + 3 = 15$

$\dfrac{3X}{4} + 3 = 15$ subtract -3
$\underline{\quad\quad -3 \quad -3}$

$\dfrac{3X}{4} = 12$

$\dfrac{3X}{4}(4) = 12\,(4)$ multiply by 4

$3X = 48$

$\dfrac{3X}{3} = \dfrac{48}{3}$ divide by 3

$$\mathbf{X = 16}$$

(VI) RATIO AND PROPORTION:

A **ratio** is composed of two numbers which are related to each other. For example, in normal saline, 0.9 grams of NaCl are contained in 100ml of water. This ratio can be written as 0.9:100 or 0.9/100 and is read 0.9 in 100. If we think about it, a ratio is really a recipe which tells us how much of an ingredient is contained in a specific volume or weight. For example, Valium injection is available in a concentration of 10mg per 2ml, which can be represented as 10mg:2ml or 10mg/2ml. This ratio (recipe) tells us that the manufacturer produced this medication by placing 10mg of Valium in each 2ml of solution.

A **proportion** consists of two ratios separated by an equal sign which indicates that the two ratios are equal.

$$10:2 = 20:4$$

This is a simple proportion and using our previous drug concentration example we can mentally verify that the ratios are indeed equal and the proportion is true.

$$10mg:2ml = 20mg:4ml$$

The numbers on the ends (10,4) of the proportion are called the extremes while the numbers in the middle of the proportion (2,20) are called the means. In a true proportion, the product of the means is equal to the product of the extremes. In the example above 10 times 4 is equal to 2 times 20 and therefore we have proven that equal ratios provide us with a true proportion.

This can also be represented in the following manner:

$$\frac{10mg}{2ml} = \frac{20mg}{4ml}$$

The first and last terms of the proportion are the extremes while the middle terms are the means. This process is also referred to as **cross multiplication**.

$$10mg \times 4ml = 20mg \times 2ml$$

$$40 = 40$$

If one quantity is unknown, the equation may be solved by substituting X for the unknown and solving for X as we have learned.

    example: If Valium injection is available in a concentration of 10mg per 2ml, how many mgs are contained in 4ml of the solution?

SOLUTION: $\dfrac{10mg}{2ml} = \dfrac{Xmg}{4ml}$

2X = 10 x 4 CROSS MULTIPLY

$$\frac{2X}{2} = \frac{40}{2}$$ SOLVE FOR X

X = 20mg

We must realize that in order for this to be a true proportion the units of each ratio must be in the same order. Therefore, if we set up the ratio on the left side as mg/ml, the ratio on the right side must be in the same order, mg/ml. Many students have problems determining where in the proportion each bit of information is placed. The following 3 step method will make this process easy.

example: If Demerol injection is available in a concentration of 25mg per ml, how many mg will be contained in 3ml?

$$\_\_\_\_\_ = \_\_\_\_\_$$

STEP 1: Place the only known ratio (recipe) in this problem on the left side of the proportion. (HINT: There is only one given ratio in this problem)

$$\frac{25mg}{1ml} = \_\_\_\_\_$$

STEP 2: Transfer the units from the ratio on the left side of the proportion to the ratio on the right side of the proportion.

$$\frac{25mg}{1ml} = \frac{mg}{ml}$$

STEP 3: Go back to the original question and fill in the right side of the proportion. That is, how many mg (X is then placed next to mg in the upper right side of the proportion) will be contained in 3ml (place a 3 in front of ml in the lower right side of the proportion) and SOLVE FOR X.

$$\frac{25mg}{1ml} = \frac{Xmg}{3\ ml}$$ CROSS MULTIPLY

X x 1 = 3 x 25   SOLVE FOR X

X = 3 x 25

X = 75mg

Sometimes, STEP 1 is cryptic, which means that the only given ratio in the question is not obvious. In some problems, the student must use their knowledge to extract a given ratio or recipe. For example, knowing that normal saline contains 0.9gm of NaCl per 100ml will give us the given ratio.

example: How many grams of NaCl are contained in 500ml of NS?

$$\frac{\quad\quad}{} = \frac{\quad\quad}{}$$

STEP 1: Look for the only given ratio and place it on the left side of the proportion. (HINT: The given ratio is NS because it contains 0.9gm NaCl in 100ml of water)

$$\frac{0.9gm}{100ml} = \frac{\quad\quad}{}$$

STEP 2: Transfer units.

$$\frac{0.9gm}{100ml} = \frac{gm}{ml}$$

STEP 3: Re-read the question to fill in the right side of the proportion.

$$\frac{0.9gm}{100ml} = \frac{Xgm}{500ml}$$

$$100X = 450$$

$$X = 4.5gm$$

(V) PERCENTAGE PREPARATIONS:

Percent (%) means "per cente" or parts per hundred. When solids are dissolved in liquids, the solid is called the "solute" and the liquid is called the "solvent". When a liquid is mixed with another liquid, the liquid present in smaller quantity is designated the "solute" while the greater quantity of liquid is the "solvent". Percentage concentrations of pharmaceutical preparations may be one of three types:

   1) *Percent weight-in-weight (w/w)* = expresses the number of grams of solute in 100 grams of product. Zinc oxide ointment contains 20% zinc oxide in white ointment. This means that each 100 grams of ointment will contain 20 grams of zinc oxide. If this preparation was being compounded in the pharmacy, 20 grams of zinc oxide would be incorporated into 80 grams of white ointment, for a total weight of 100 grams.

   2) *Percent weight-in-volume (w/v)* = expresses the number of grams of solute in 100ml of solution. A 20% potassium chloride solution will contain 20 grams of potassium chloride in each 100ml of solution.

   3) *Percent volume-in-volume (v/v)* = expresses the number of milliliters of a liquid contained in each 100ml of solution. 95% alcohol contains 95ml of alcohol in each 100ml of solution.

RULE: When asked to calculate the percentage strength of a preparation, just set the concentration equal to X/100.

example: If 250gm of an ointment contains 7.5gm of hydrocortisone, what is the percentage strength (w/w) of this ointment?

$$\_\_\_\_ = \frac{X}{100}$$

$$\frac{\_\_\_\_\_}{250 \text{ gm}} = \frac{X}{100}$$

$$250X = 750$$

$$\frac{250}{250} = \frac{750}{250}$$

X = 3%

example: How many grams of zinc oxide are needed to prepare 750 gm of a 20% zinc oxide ointment?

STEP 1: Known ratio on left $\dfrac{20gm}{100gm}$ = _____

···➔

STEP 2: Transfer units $\dfrac{20gm}{100gm}$ = $\dfrac{\_\_\_\_gm}{gm}$

···➔

STEP 3: Fill in right side $\dfrac{20gm}{100gm}$ = $\dfrac{Xgm}{750gm}$ CROSS MULTIPLY

SOLVE FOR X: 100X = 15000

X = 150gm

example: How many grams of zinc chloride are needed to prepare 1500ml of a 1:50 solution?

STEP 1: Known ratio on left $\dfrac{1gm}{50ml}$ =_____

···➔

STEP 2: Transfer units $\dfrac{1gm}{50ml}$ = $\dfrac{\_\_\_gm}{ml}$

···➔

STEP 3: Fill in right side

$$\frac{1gm}{50ml} = \frac{Xgm}{1500ml} \quad \text{CROSS MULTIPLY}$$

SOLVE FOR X: 50X = 1500

X = 30gm

(VI) TEMPERATURE CONVERSION

Both Fahrenheit and Centigrade temperatures are commonly used in pharmacy practice. The pharmacy technician must be able to convert
from one scale of measurement to the other.

  1) **Centigrade** = is calibrated so that the freezing point of water is 0 degrees and the boiling point of water is 100 degrees.

  2) **Fahrenheit** = is calibrated so that the freezing point of water is 32 degrees and the boiling point of water is 212 degrees.

To convert a temperature from one scale to the other, the following formula is used:

9 x C degrees = (5 x F degrees) - 160

example: Convert 10 degrees Centigrade to Fahrenheit.
9 x 10 = 5F - 160

$$90 = 5F - 160$$
$$\underline{+160 = \quad + 160}$$
$$250 = 5F$$

$$\frac{250}{5} = \frac{5F}{5}$$

F = 50

example: Convert 80 degrees Fahrenheit to Centigrade.

9 X C = (5 x 80) - 160

9C = 240

$$\frac{9C}{9} = \frac{240}{9}$$

C = 26.6

104

VII) DOSAGE CALCULATIONS:

To determine the number of doses, quantity of each dose, or the size of each dose to be dispensed, use the following formula:

Number of doses = $\dfrac{\text{Total amount}}{\text{Size of each dose}}$

example: How many doses are contained in 2gm, if the dosage is 50mg?

$$\text{Number of doses} = \frac{2000mg}{50mg}$$

Number of doses = 40

example: What dosage should be administered if 30gm of a medication is to be divided into 20 doses?

$$20 \text{ doses} = \frac{30gm}{X}$$

$$20X = 30gm$$

$$\frac{20X}{20} = \frac{30gm}{20}$$

X = 1.5gm per dose

example: Calculate the amount of syrup to be dispensed to provide 20 doses (qid x 5 days) of 5ml per dose?

$$20 = \frac{X}{5ml}$$

X = 100ml

(VIII) CHILDREN'S DOSES:

Several formulas may be used to estimate doses for children or infants. The following two formulas are based on the normal adult dose.

Clark's Rule: $\dfrac{\text{weight of child (lbs)}}{150} \times \text{adult dose} = \text{child's dose}$

Young's Rule: $\dfrac{\text{child's age (yrs)}}{\text{child's age} + 12} \times \text{adult dose} = \text{child's dose}$

Note: Since Clark's Rule is based on the weight of the child, it is more widely used.

The most accurate method of determining dosages for children based on adult dosages is the **Body Surface Area** method. The body surface area (BSA) for the child is determined from a nomogram that calculates BSA from the weight and size of the child. The formula used with this method is:

Child's dose = $\dfrac{\text{child's BSA}}{1.73}$ x adult dose

(IX) DILUTION OF STOCK SOLUTIONS:

Concentrated stock solutions may be used to prepare more dilute solutions and is an important aspect of pharmacy practice. The following formula should be used for diluting stock solutions:

quantity x strength = quantity x strength

$$Q1 \ \times \ S1 \ = \ Q2 \ \times \ S2$$

Q1 = weight or volume of stock solution

S1 = strength of stock solution

Q2 = weight or volume of desired solution

S2 = strength of desired solution

example: How many grams of a 1% hydrocortisone cream can be made from 240gm of 2.5% hydrocortisone cream?

$$Q1 \times S1 \ = \ Q2 \times S2$$

$$240gm \times 2.5\% \ = \ Xgm \times 1\%$$

$$240 \times .025 = X \times .01$$

$$6 = .01X$$
$$\frac{6}{.01} = \frac{.01X}{.01}$$

X = 600gm

ALLIGATION

If the desired percentage concentration of a solution, ointment or cream required to fill a prescription or medication order is not available, it can be compounded by mixing stronger and weaker components to obtain the desired strength. This method is referred to as "alligation alternate" and is used to determine the number of "parts" or "proportions" of each component used to prepare the specific strength.

The following steps review this method:

STEP 1: Place a large "X" in the center of your paper. The upper and lower left 2 corners of the "X" are reserved for the percentages of components being used. The upper left corner reflects the higher strength while the lower left corner reflects the lower strength concentration being used. The middle section of the "X" is reserved for the desired strength.

PERCENTAGE   **PARTS**

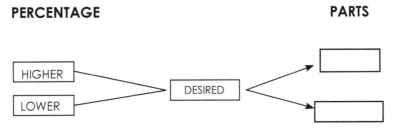

STEP 2: The upper and lower right corners of the "X" are derived by calculating the difference between the higher and desired strength which is placed in the lower right corner of the "X" and the difference between the lower and desired strength which is placed in the upper right corner of the "X". The total number of parts is then calculated.

PERCENTAGE   **PARTS**

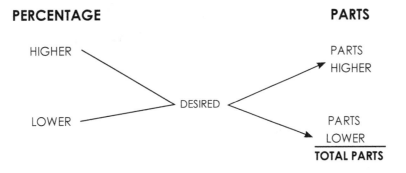

STEP 3: Once the proportional parts have been determined, the quantities of the higher and lower strength preparation may be calculated by setting each equal to x divided by the total quantity of preparation to be compounded.

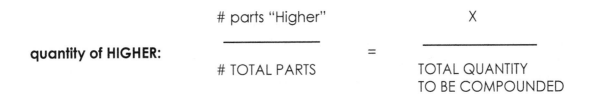

$$\textbf{quantity of HIGHER:} \quad \frac{\# \text{ parts ``Higher''}}{\# \text{ TOTAL PARTS}} = \frac{X}{\text{TOTAL QUANTITY TO BE COMPOUNDED}}$$

	# parts "Lower"		X
quantity of LOWER:	————————	=	————————
	# total parts		TOTAL QUANTITY TO BE COMPOUNDED

example: What quantity of a 70% dextrose solution must be mixed with a 20% dextrose solution to obtain 1liter (1000ml) of a 35% dextrose solution?

STEP 1:

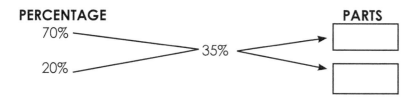

STEP 2:

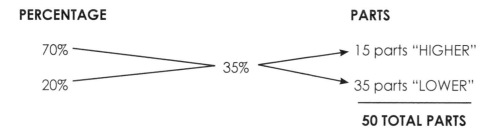

STEP 3:

70%: $\dfrac{15}{50} = \dfrac{X}{1000ml}$ **X = 300 ml**

20%: $\dfrac{35}{50} = \dfrac{X}{1000ml}$ **X = 700 ml**

To compound this prescription, 300ml of 70% dextrose is added to 700ml of 20% dextrose to make a total of 1 liter of a 35% dextrose solution.

HINTS:
1) If water or an ointment base containing no drug entity is used as the lower component then 0 (zero) is placed in the lower left corner of the "X".
2) The total of both components together must add up to the total quantity required for the prescription order.

example: 20 gms of a 7.5% zinc oxide ointment is prescribed by a dermatologist. The pharmacy has a 10% ointment and Aquaphor available in stock. How many grams of each will be required to compound this prescription?

STEP 1:

PERCENTAGE   **PARTS**

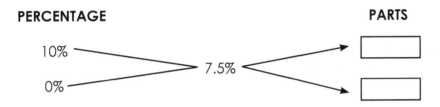

STEP 2:

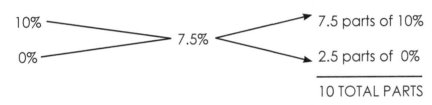

STEP 3:

10% ointment	$\dfrac{7.5}{10}$	$=$	$\dfrac{X}{20\ gm}$	**X=15gm**

Aquaphor	$\dfrac{2.5}{10}$	$=$	$\dfrac{X}{20\ gms}$	**X=5gm**

REMEMBER: Always check your answer by adding together the quantity of each component to make sure it adds up to the total quantity required.

(X) FLOW RATE CALCULATIONS

To determine the flow rate of parenteral solution, the following formula is used:

drops/minute = <u>ml of solution x number of drops/ml</u>
<u>minutes of administration (hrs x 60)</u>

example: Determine the flow rate to be used to infuse 2 liters of D5W over 12 hours if the set delivers 10 drops per ml?

$$\text{drops/minute} = \frac{2000ml \times 10gtts/ml}{12hrs \times 60min/hr}$$

$$\text{drops/minute} = \frac{20,000}{720}$$

X = 28gtts/min

(XI) INFUSION TIME CALCULATIONS

To determine the infusion time of a parenteral solution, use the following equation:

$$\text{volume of solution} \times \frac{\text{drops}}{ml} \times \frac{\text{minutes}}{\text{drops}} \times \frac{1hr}{60 min}$$

example: Determine the infusion time of 1 liter of NS if an infusion set delivering 20 drops/ml is set at 40 drops/min.

$$\frac{1000ml \times 20gtts}{ml} \times \frac{1min}{40gtts} \times \frac{1hr}{60 min} = \frac{20,000}{2400k} = \textbf{8.3 hours}$$

(XII) BUSINESS MATH IN PHARMACY PRACTICE

The essential business concepts are:

1) **OVERHEAD** - the cost of doing business.

2) **NET PROFIT** - the amount of money that remains after the cost of purchasing, handling, storing, selling of the drug. This cost is subtracted from the selling price to derive the net profit.

3) **GROSS PROFIT** - the difference between the purchase price and the selling price.

Selling Price - Purchase Price = Gross Profit

4) **MARKUP** - the difference between the purchase price and the
       selling price.

Selling Price - Purchase Price = Markup

$$\frac{Markup}{Cost} = Markup\ Rate$$

5) **DISCOUNT** - the reduced price, or a deduction from the amount due.

6) **INVENTORY** - a listing of drugs and other supplies and merchandise
       that is available for sale.

$$Average\ Inventory = \frac{(Beginning\ Inventory + Ending\ Inventory)}{2}$$

7) **TURNOVER** - the amount of inventory compared to the total annual
       purchases.

$$Turnover\ Rate = \frac{Annual\ \$\ Purchases\ (products,\ drugs,\ etc.)}{Average\ Inventory}$$

8) **DEPRECIATION** - the allowance made for the decreasing value
       of an asset.

$$Annual\ Depreciation = \frac{(Total\ Cost - Disposal\ Value)}{Estimated\ Life\ (yrs.)}$$

9) **AWP** - the average wholesale price of a drug or device.

Aquisition Cost = AWP - Discount

PRACTICE PROBLEMS

I) CONVERSIONS

1) A formula for a cough syrup contains 1/8 grain of codeine per teaspoonful. How many grams of codeine would be needed to prepare 1 quart of the cough syrup?

2) A prescription calls for 1/100 gr of atropine SO4 per capsule, with a total of 60 capsules to be compounded. How many 0.4 mg atropine SO4 tablets will be required to prepare these capsules?

3) Lanoxin Injection is available in a concentration of 0.25mg per 1 ml. How many ml of the injection will be required for a 90 microgram dose?

4) The dose of a drug is 1/15 gr/kg of body weight. If the patient weighs 165 lbs, how many milligrams of the drug should the patient receive?

5) If 50 gms of a powder is repacked into 75 unit dose packages, how many grains will each package contain?

II) CALCULATION OF DOSES

1) A child's Ceclor dose is 40mg/kg/day in 3 divided doses.
   a) If the child weighs 41 pounds, how many grams of Ceclor will the child receive daily?
   b) How many milligrams will the child receive per dose?
   c) What quantity of the 250mg/5ml suspension would be dispensed for a 10 day therapy?
   d) What directions for use should appear on the dispensing label?
    e) Which auxiliary labels should be affixed to the drug container?

2) The initial loading dose of vancomycin for infants is 30mg/kg/day.
   a) What would be the dose in milligrams, for an neonate weighing 3500 grams?
   b) How many milliliters of an injection containing 500mg/25ml should be used to administer this dose?

3) How many grams of acetaminophen will a 50 pound patient receive in two successive days at a dosage of 10mg/kg/dose every 4 hours?

4) Naldecon Pediatric Drops contain 270mg of pseudoephedrine per fluid ounce. How many milligrams of the drug would be administered to a child who is receiving a 1/4 ml dose?

III) *PERCENTAGE + RATIO STRENGTH*

1) How many grams of hydrocortisone will be found in 1 lb of a 2.5% HC cream?

2) What is the percentage of hydrocortisone in a product containing 1.5 gms of hydrocortisone in 120 gms of cream?

3) If 250 ml of 1:400 (v/v) solution is diluted to 1 liter, what will be the resultant percentage strength?

4) If 500 ml of a 30% (w/v) is diluted to 2 liters, what is the ratio strength of the dilution?

5) A solution contains 4000mg of a drug in 1 pint;
      a) What is the % (w/v) of the solution?
      b) What is the ratio strength of the solution?
      c) What is the mg/ml concentration of the solution?

IV) DILUTION + CONCENTRATION

1) How many ml of a 1:100 (w/v) stock solution must be used to prepare 2 liters of a 1:3000 (w/v) solution?

2) How many ml of normal saline solution (0.9%) may be prepared from 500 ml of a 30% (w/v) stock solution?

3) How many grams of 10% ointment should be mixed with a 2% ointment to make 1/2 lb of a 5 % ointment?

4) How many ml of 95% ethyl alcohol should be mixed with water to make 1.5 liters of a 30% ethanol solution?

5) A prescription calls for 0.0025g of atropine sulfate. How much of a 1:10 stock powder must be used for this Rx?

V) *FLOW RATE + INFUSION TIME*
1) What is the flow rate for 50 ml of D5W containing 100mg of minocycline infused over 1 hour if the administration set is calibrated to deliver 15 drops per ml?

2) A physician orders 10 units of insulin to be mixed in 1 liter of D5W to be administered over a 6 hour period;
      a) How many drops per minute should be administered if the set is calibrated to deliver 20 drops per ml?
      b) How much insulin will be delivered in the first 45 minutes of the infusion?

3) A piggyback containing 1 gm of kefzol in 100 ml of D5W is to be infused at a flow rate of 50 gtts/min and the administration set is calibrated to deliver 15 gtts/ml. How long will it take to administer the entire piggyback?

4) An infant is to receive 25 ml of a solution at 25 gtts/min. If the set is calibrated to deliver 60 gtts/ml, how long will it take to deliver this solution?

5) 800 ml of Lactated Ringers has been ordered to be administered over a 6 hour period. If the set has been calibrated to deliver 10 gtts/ml, at what flow rate should this IV be administered?

VI) BUSINESS MATH

1) The AWP for nystatin suspension is $8.95 per 60ml bottle. If the markup is 12% and a $7.50 dispensing fee is added, what is the selling price of this medication?

2) The AWP for for generic Zantac 150mg is $30.37 per pack of 24 tablets. If the pharmacy retails it for $39.95, what is the markup rate for this drug?

3) A pharmacy does quarterly inventory and has an average inventory value of $125,000. Annual purchases are $350,000. What is the turnover rate?

4) The discount on a wholesaler invoice of $3300 is 8%/15, net 30. If the account is paid in full after 14 days, what is the total discounted purchase price of this invoice?

5) If the cash discount on a $5500 wholesaler invoice is $385, what is the % discount for this invoice?

SEE NEXT PAGE FOR COMPLETE ANSWERS

ANSWERS

I) CONVERSIONS

1) Total amount for Rx: 0.125gr/5ml = Xgr/946ml X = 23.65gr
   Convert gr to gm: 1gm/15.4gr = Xgm/23.65gr
   X = 1.53gm of codeine

2) Total amount for Rx: 0.01gr/1 cap = Xgr/60 caps X = 0.6gr
   Convert gr to mg : 1gr/65mg = 0.6gr/Xmg X = 39mg
   Number of 0.4mg tabs: X = 39mg/0.4mg
   X = 97.5 tablets of atropine

3) Change micrograms to mg: 90mcg = 0.09mg
   Calculate volume needed: 0.25mg/1ml = 0.09mg/Xml
   X = 0.36ml of Lanoxin Inj.

4) Convert lbs to kg: 1kg/2.2lbs = Xkg/165 X = 75kg
   Calculate dose: 0.066gr/1kg = X/75kg x = 4.95gr
   Convert gr to mg: 1gr/65mg = 4.95gr/Xmg
   X = 321.75mg of drug

5) Change gm to gr: 1gm/15.4gr = 50gm/Xgr X = 770gr
   Divide into U/D packages: X = 770gr/75packages
   X = 10.26gr per U/D pack

II) CALCULATION OF DOSES

1a) Convert lb to kg: 1kg/2.2lb = Xkg/41lb X = 18.63kg
   Calculate total dose: 40mg/1kg = Xmg/18.63kg X = 745.2mg
   Convert mg to gm:
   X = 0.745gm Ceclor per day

1b) Divide mg dose by 3: X = 745mg/3
   X = 248.4mg (250mg) of Ceclor per dose

1c) Calculate total volume: 5ml x 3 doses per day x 10 days
   X = 150ml of Ceclor

1d) **Take one teaspoonful (5ml) by mouth 3 times daily for 10 days**

1e) **SHAKE WELL, REFRIGERATE, DISCARD AFTER 14 DAYS,
   FINISH ALL MEDICATION**

2a) Convert gm to kg: 3500gm = 3.5kg
   Calculate dose: 30mg/1kg = Xmg/3.5kg
   X = 105mg of vancomycin per day

2b) Calculate volume of IV: 500mg/25ml = 105mg/Xml
   X = 5.25ml of IV solution

3) Convert lb to kg: 1kg/2.2lb = Xkg/50lb X = 22.7kg
   Calculate single dose: 10mg/kg = Xmg/22.7kg X = 227.2mg
   Calculate 2 days dose: 227.2mg x 6 doses per day x 2 days
      X = 2.72gm of APAP in 2 days

4) Calculate dose: 270mg/30ml = Xmg/0.25ml
      X = 2.25mg per 1/4ml

III) *PERCENTAGE + RATIO STRENGTH*
1) Convert lb to gm: 1lb = 454gm
   Calculate total drug: 2.5gm/100gm = Xgm/454gm
      X = 11.35gm HC in one lb

2) Percentage: X/100
   Calculate %: 1.5gm/120gm = Xgm/100gm
      X = 1.25%

3) Calculate amount of drug in original solution: 1gm/400ml = Xgm/250ml
      X = 0.625gm
   Dilute and calculate %: 0.625gm/1000ml = X/100
      X = 0.0625% after dilution

4) Ratio strength: 1/X
   Calculate amount of drug in original solution: 30gm/100ml = Xgm/500ml
      X = 150gm
   Dilute and ratio strength: 150gm/2000ml = 1/X dilution
      X = 3:40 resultant ratio strength

5a) Calculate %: 4gm/473ml = X/100
      X = 0.84%

5b) Set equal to 1/X: 4gm/473ml = 1/X
      X = 1 : 118 ratio strength

5c) Set equal to X/1: 4000mg/473ml = Xmg/1ml
      X = 8.45mg/1ml

IV) *DILUTION + CONCENTRATION*
1) Use the following formula: Q1 x S1 = Q2 x S2 where Q is the quantity and S
   is the strength of each solution.
   Xml x 1/100 = 2000ml x 1/3000
   X/100 = 2000/3000
      X = 66.6ml of 1:100 (w/v) stock solution

2) Use the following formula: Q1 x S1 = Q2 x S2
   Xml x 0.9/100 = 500ml x 30/100
   0.9x/100 = 15000/100
      X = 16666.6ml or 16.6 liters of NS

3) Alligation alternate should be used to calculate this problem:
   # parts of 10% ointment: 3 parts/8 total parts
   # parts of 2% ointment: 5 parts/8 total parts
   To make 1/2 lb; quantity of 10% ointment: 3/8 = X/227
   X = 85.1gm of 10% ointment
   quantity of 2 % ointment: 5/8 = x/227
   X = 141.9gm of 2% ointment
   TOTAL = 85.1gm + 141.9gm = 227gm = 1/2 pound

4) Alligation alternate should be used to calculate this problem:
   # parts of 95% ethanol: 30 parts/95 total parts
   # parts of water (0%) : 65 parts/95 total parts
   To make 1500ml;
   quantity of 95% ethanol: 30/95 = X/1500
   X = 474ml of 95% ethanol
   quantity of water (0%) : 65/95 = X/1500
   X = 1026ml of water

5) 25ml

V) FLOW RATE + INFUSION TIME

1) $\dfrac{50ml \times 15gtts/ml}{60min}$ = **12.5gtts/min**

2) a. $\dfrac{100ml \times 20gtts/ml}{360\ min}$ = **55.5gtts/min**

   b. 10units/360min = Xunits/45min **X = 1.25units of insulin**

3) 100ml x $\dfrac{15gtts}{1ml}$ x $\dfrac{1min}{50gtts}$ x $\dfrac{1hr}{60min}$ = **1/2 hour or 30 minutes**

4) 25ml x $\dfrac{60gtts}{1ml}$ x $\dfrac{1min}{25gtts}$ x $\dfrac{1hr}{60min}$ = **1 hour or 60 minutes**

5) $\dfrac{800ml \times 10gtts/ml}{360min}$ = **22.2gtts/min**

VI) BUSINESS MATH

1) $8.95 x 0.12 = $1.07
   $8.95 + $1.07 + $7.50 = **$17.52 per 60ml bottle of nystatin suspension**

2) Markup = $39.95 - $30.37 = $9.58
   $\dfrac{\$9.58}{\$30.37}$ = 0.32 x 100 = **32% Markup**

3) $\dfrac{\$350,000}{\$125,000}$ = **2.8 Turnover Rate**

4) 8%/15, means that if the invoice is paid within 15 days,
an 8% discount be applied. If not paid within 15 days then the full amount
must be paid within 30 days. In this example the discount will apply
since it is being paid after 14 days.

$3300 x 0.08 = $264 discount
$3300 - $264 = **$3036 Total Discounted Purchase Price**

5) $\dfrac{\$385}{\$5500}$ = 0.07 x100 = **7% discount**

SECTION 7A: TASK EVALUATIONS - RETAIL

The pharmacy technician must be competent in the following tasks when practicing in the retail setting. This section will attempt to break down each task into components so that the pharmacy technician can understand what functions may be expected.

1) PURCHASING AND INVENTORY CONTROL:
   a) Understands inventory goals including turnover rate, minimum quantity needed to reorder and methods required for low inventory. A well stocked pharmacy consists of sufficient stock for proper dispensing without shortages.
   b) Can differentiate the source of each medication . "Direct" ordering is the purchasing of drugs directly from the manufacturer. This direct price usually reflects the lowest price for a drug, but since many companies will not sell directly to the retailer, many drugs must be purchased from the "Wholesaler". The wholesale price is usually about 10% higher than the direct price but wholesalers offer a wider variety of products, services and discounts.
   c) Utilizes a "reorder list" - which is the notation in a "want book" of the product to be ordered. Many retail institutions have separate lists for products to be ordered depending on the source from where they are purchased. Many wholesalers provide the pharmacy with hand held reorder computers (TELZON) to transmit these reorder lists via phone modem.
   d) Performs purchasing process - Knows the process of transmitting "reorder lists" via phone modem and computer.
   e) Properly checks and reorders inventory.
   f) "Checks-in" orders properly - notifies the person in charge of ordering of backorders (drugs that the supplier is out of stock), checks for shortages, damaged items, and the correctness of price of each item ordered.
   g) Stocks meds correctly - places refrigerated items in the refrigerator, properly rotates stock by placing the product with the shortest expiration date first and restocks items in their correct place.
   h) Handles returns and credits properly - understands the proper procedures and documentation required for returning drugs for credit.
   i) Understands procedure for "drug recalls".
   j) Checks for expired meds in inventory - each time a medication is handled the expiration date is checked. If med is expired, knows proper procedure for return.
   k) Can retrieve medications from stock.
   l) Monitors proper drug storage conditions - as outlined by the USP-NF with
   m) Understands the process of borrowing meds - commonly referred to as "KOWing" from other pharmacies, know which pharmacies will provide this service for your pharmacy.

2) ADMINISTRATIVE TASKS - POLICIES AND PROCEDURES:

a) Understands basic policy and procedures.
b) Can differentiate between pharmacist and tech responsibilities - for both professional practice and liability.
c) Respects patient confidentiality - and understands the liability associated with breach of confidentiality.
d) Ability to interact with other professionals.
e) Ability to interact with the consumer.
f) Displays proper phone etiquette.
g) Complies with professional and legal standards.
h) Understands workload priorities - when multiple tasks are required, the pharmacy technician must prioritize tasks correctly.
i) Knows hours of business scheduling.

3) PRESCRIPTION PROCESSING - DISPENSING:

a) Knows normal Rx workload flow.
b) Obtains proper information for patient profile - including patient data (name, address, phone # and age), medical history and diagnosis, method of payment (private vs third party insurance), allergies and contraindications, and type of container to be dispensed (childproof vs easy-open).
c) Determines if prescription is valid and properly written by prescriber.
d) Interprets all aspects of prescription correctly.
e) Enters order into computer properly.
f) Correctly retrieves refill prescription from files.
g) Knows trade and generic names of medications.
h) Fills order correctly.
i) Correctly completes proper records.
j) Knows refill status for all medications.
k) Knows how to reconstitute oral powders.
l) Affixes appropriate auxiliary labels to container.
m) Correctly bills patient for Rx - by understanding fee structures for private billing, insurance co-pays, public assistance and employee discounts.
n) Completes charge and cash transactions correctly.
o) Correctly files prescriptions - CII, CIII-CIV and non-controlled Rx's.
p) Understands various routes of drug administration - including ophthalmic, otic, vaginal, rectal, nasal and transdermal patches. Also must be able to differentiate between long-acting and immediate acting dosage forms.
q) Can correctly calculate doses and units to be dispensed.
r) Knows when to substitute for generic equivalents.
s) Maintains an organized, clean work area.
t) Properly uses the cash register.

4) THIRD PARTY INSURANCE:

a) Identifies proper prescription coverages.
b) Differentiates correctly among prescription plans.
c) Checks patient and dependent eligibility prior to filling the prescription.
d) Fills prescription according to plan coverage.
e) Bills co-pay correctly.
 f) Runs computerized third party payment forms.

5) COMPUTER SYSTEMS:

a) Understands technician's computer responsibilities.
b) Correctly performs order entry on the computer.
c) Modifies existing orders when needed.
d) Generates proper label.
e) Reviews patient profile properly - including diagnosis, allergies, drug interactions and contraindications.
 f) Monitors inventory control - if applicable.

6) MEDICAL SUPPLIES:

a) Familiar with:
- vaporizers and humidifiers
- thermometers;
    rectal, oral, otic, basal and digital.
- eye irrigation cups
- nasal syringes;
    infant, children's and adult.
- otic syringes
- syringes
- heating pads;
    moist and dry.
- enemas;
    pediatric, children's and adult.
- douches
- nebulizers
- glucometers
- I.D. bracelets

7) SURGICAL SUPPLIES:

a) Familiar with:
- wheelchairs
- walkers
- bedpans and urinals
- disposable underpads
- ostomy supplies
- canes and crutches
- braces

8) CONTROLLED SUBSTANCES:

a) Knows federal, state and local pharmacy laws.
b) Understands all schedules of controlled substances.
c) Knows the process of ordering CII medications.
d) Fills prescription according to plan coverage.
e) Bills co-pay correctly.
f) Runs computerized third party payment forms.
e) Knows procedure for storage of controlled drugs.
f) Maintains on-going inventory of controlled drugs.
g) Can identify a fraudulent prescription.
h) Knows procedure for Schedule V over-the-counter drugs, where applicable.
i) Knows refill procedures for all schedules.
j) Understands how/where to file controlled drugs.

9) OTC MEDICATIONS:

a) Understands the use for major OTC products.
b) Can locate OTC products for the consumer.

10) MISCELLANEOUS SERVICES:

a) Can discuss the use of the following:
- deliveries
- patient profiles
- income tax receipts
- insurance receipts
- customer charges
b) Know how to bill supplies to physicians' offices.

SECTION 7B: TASK EVALUATIONS - INSTITUTIONAL

The pharmacy technician must be competent in the following tasks when practicing in the institutional setting. This section will attempt to break down each task into components so that the pharmacy technician can understand what functions must be mastered.

1) ADMINISTRATIVE TASKS - POLICY AND PROCEDURES:
a) Understands basic policy and procedures.
b) Knows organizational chart (institution and pharmacy).
c) Understands technician responsibility and liability.
d) Understands disciplinary action policy.
e) Respects patient confidentiality.
f) Ability to interact with professionals/peers.
g) Displays proper phone etiquette.
h) Complies with legal and professional standards.
i) Understands workload priorities.
j) Understands pharmacy's relationship to other departments.
k) Knowledgeable about JCAHO requirements.

2) PURCHASING AND INVENTORY CONTROL:
a) Understands inventory goals (turn-over rate, min. levels, reorders)
b) Differentiates between direct vs wholesalers.
c) Utilizes a reorder list (i.e. want book).
d) Performs purchasing process (phone, modem).
e) Properly checks and reorders inventory.
f) Completes inventory delivery (checks for backorders, shortages, damages, correct price).
g) Stocks meds correctly (rotation of stock, generic vs trade name, by manufacturer, in refrigerator).
h) Differentiates between non-formulary and formulary meds.
i) Knows procedures for handling non-formulary meds.
j) Knows how to handle returns and credits.
k) Verifies correctness of price via invoice.
l) Knows procedure on drug recalls.
m) Knows procedure on expired medication.
n) Generates inventory reports.
o) Properly handles controlled substances inventory.
p) Knows procedure for interdepartmental ordering.
q) Can retrieve meds from stock as needed.
r) Identifies drugs requiring special storage.
s) Files invoices in compliance with the law.

3) DISPENSING:

a) Understands institution drug delivery system (i.e. decentralized, unit dose, traditional).
b) Knows normal order flow.
c) Properly identifies med order on physician order sheet.
d) Interprets med order correctly.
e) Understands handling of STATS, ASAP drugs.
f) Enters order correctly (via computer/manual).
g) Knows trade/generic names.
h) Fills order correctly.
i) Understands different types of drug packages (multi- dose, single dose, aerosols/sprays, tubes)
j) Labels drug correctly.
k) Follows "final check" system.
l) Identifies different delivery systems.
m) Distributes meds to pts. and other hospital depts.
n) Properly prepares a patient profile.
o) Understands various routes of drug administration.
p) Can identify improper dosing.
q) Properly fills unit dose cassettes from pick list.
r) Exchanges unit dose carts correctly.
s) Understands institution's generic drug policy.
t) Reconstitutes pharmaceuticals when necessary.
u) Correctly calculates doses when necessary.
v) Prices meds/services according to policy.
w) Uses auxiliary labels appropriately.
x) Refers appropriate problems to pharmacist.
y) Knows procedure for dispensing controlled substances.
z) Properly retrieves and files records.

4) PREPACKAGING:

a) Identifies proper prepackaging equipment.
b) Properly assembles and uses unit dose equipment.
c) Properly cleans and stores unit dose equipment.
d) Selects correct medication for prepackaging.
e) Knows proper stability information for prepackaging.
f) Accurately performs calculations and measurements when necessary.
g) Completes worksheet records (logs of lot numbers, mfg., weights, volumes).
h) Correct procedures for mixing and preparing formulations.
i) Properly selects and prepares containers and closures.
j) Uses correct packaging technique.
k) Correctly selects and prepares label for UD meds.
l) Identifies proper drug storage requirements (light sensitivity, refrigeration)
m) Knows requirements for labeling on prepackaged products.
n) Knows how to prevent contamination of UD meds.
o) Knows how to prepare "oral suspensions".
p) Knows procedure for drug recalls.
q) Identifies quality control procedures.

5) COMPUTERS:
a) Understands technician's computer responsibilities.
b) Correctly performs order entry on a computer.
c) Modifies existing orders when necessary.
d) Performs patient admissions, transfers and discharges on the computer.
e) Performs label printing on the computer.
f) Performs generation of:
- pick list
- med administration record
- medication profile
- updated/modified list
g) Properly uses computer to:
- review patient diagnosis
- review allergies/sensitivities
- monitor drug interactions
- monitor inventory control - bill/credit patients

6) INTRAVENOUS ADMIXTURES:
a) Knows principles of aseptic technique.
b) Knows procedures for functioning in laminar flow hood (vertical and horizontal).
c) Proper interpretation of IV orders.
d) Enters IV order onto pt. profile when necessary.
e) Correctly performs IV calculations.
f) Properly selects the needed ingredients.
g) Correctly measures the ingredients.
h) Properly labels the IV product.
i) Identifies proper stability information.
j) Can retrieve IV incompatibility information when necessary.
k) Knows IV storage requirements.
l) Maintains quality control and uses proper records for documentation.
m) Identifies various types of drug packages/containers (large volume, small volume, multidose, single dose).
n) Knows policy/procedure for handling chemotherapy.
o) Knows how to dispose of chemo.
p) Identify different IV systems:
- frozen
- fast-pak
- ADD-vantage
- premixtures
- syringe pumps
- traditional dilution
q) Knows how to use IV compounders (i.e. Automix)
r) Familiar with different IV administration sets.
s) Properly identifies which IV pump to use and when.
t) Demonstrates proper technique for aseptic withdrawal of contents from a rubber capped vial and a glass ampule.
u) Utilizes proper procedure for IV antibiotic reconstitution.
v) Knows institution's procedure on IV infiltration.

w) Correctly calculates the IV flow rate.
x) Correctly compounds a TPN admixture.
y) Correctly delivers IV solutions and stores it properly.
z) Identifies different routes of parenteral administration.
- Knows different types of syringes.
- Knows different types of needles.
- Knows different routes of parenteral administration.

7) CONTROLLED SUBSTANCES:
a) Knows federal, state and local pharmacy laws.
b) Discusses all schedules of controlled substances.
c) Knows procedure for special storage conditions for controlled substances.
d) Knows proper inventory control for controlled substances.
e) Knows procedure for Schedule V over-the-counter drugs.
f) Knows when to conduct inventory.
g) Maintains records for proper controlled substance counts.
h) Knows regulations governing the dispensing of syringes.
i) Discusses refill information for all Schedules.

8) FLOOR STOCK:
a) Knows replacement policy for nursing units stock meds.
b) Familiar with floor stock lists.
c) Knows how to perform a nursing station inspection.
d) Fills floor stock orders.
e) Manufactures stock solutions
- use of worksheets
- identify procedure used

9) INFORMATION SYSTEMS:
a) Utilizes computerized information systems (Microdex, CD-ROM, modem)
b) Familiar with reference books that have stability data included.
c) Identifies procedure for answering questions from:
- physicians
- nurses
- healthcare professionals
- general public
d) Familiar with basic pharmacy texts.
e) Identifies sources available (i.e. textbooks, journals, subscription services, retrieval system)
f) Identifies phone numbers of drug information and poison control centers.
g) Locates information sources.
h) Retrieves information.

10) MISCELLANEOUS:
   a) Identify special record keeping of:
      - investigational drugs
      - non-formulary drugs
   b) Proper selection of correct measuring device when compounding.
   c) Compounds enteral products.
   d) Identifies "home med" policy.
   e) Reviews emergency medication policy when the pharmacy is closed.
   f) Understands JCAHO requirements.
   g) Provides data retrieval for drug utilization evaluation programs.
   h) Replaces ER medications.
   i) Replaces OR medications.
   j) Replaces stock to code boxes and crash carts.

SECTION 8: CERTIFICATION-TYPE QUESTIONS

The National Certification Examination contains 100 multiple choice questions. Be sure to bring a non-programmable calculator to the exam and use the hints indicated at the beginning of the text. The content and trends of the following certification-type questions have been asked on previous certification examinations.

PRACTICE EXAM #1

1) When dispensing Ventolin Inhaler, how often must the Patient Package Insert (PPI) be included with the drug product?
   a) at the time the original Rx is dispensed
   b) every time the prescription is dispensed
   c) every other time that the prescription is dispensed
   d) it should never be dispensed with the prescription

2) A prescription is written for Penicillin VK 250mg tabs po qid for 10 days. If the patient cannot swallow tablets and requests a liquid dosage form, what volume of 250mg/ 5ml suspension should be dispensed?
   a) 50ml
   b) 100ml
   c) 150ml
   d) 200ml

3) Which drug requires a follow-up "cover" prescription when dispensed as a verbal order?
   a) phenobarbital
   b) atenolol
   c) buspirone
   d) procainamide

4) The expiration date on a bottle of Cipro 500mg tablets states 4/13. When does this drug expire?
   a) midnight 3/31/13
   b) midnight 4/1/13
   c) midnight 4/30/13
   d) midnight 5/1/13

5) What volume of a 2% erythromycin solution can be made from 15gms of erythromycin powder?
   a) 250ml
   b) 500ml
   c) 750ml
   d) 1000ml

6) The middle set of digits in a National Drug Code (NDC) number represents:
    a) the manufacturer
    b) the product size
    c) the cost of the product
    d) the product strength and dosage form

7) Estraderm is available in which dosage form?
    a) oral
    b) patch
    c) topical cream
    d) IV

8) Pseudoephedrine, a common ingredient in cold preparations, is contraindicated in which of the following disease states?
    a) hypertension
    b) diabetes
    c) constipation
    d) cancer

9) Which drug agency is responsible to regulate medical devices?
    a) EPA
    b) DEA
    c) OSHA
    d) FDA

10) If Domeboro tablets are received from the wholesaler, where should they be stocked?
    a) next to Dolobid 500mg tablets
    b) where the Bacitracin ointment is stored
    c) with Mycostatin vaginal suppositories
    d) in the refrigerator with EES suspension

11) Which of the following medications may not be crushed?
    a) Ecotrin 325mg
    b) Fiorinal
    c) Inderal 10mg
    d) Robaxin 500mg

12) The directions for use of a medication is " i sl prn." The meaning of "sl" is:
    a) into the skin
    b) under the tongue
    c) into the muscle
    d) into the right eye

13) What type of prescription balance must be used for compounding 120gms of a 1% topical antifungal cream?
   a) class A prescription balance
   b) class B prescription balance
   c) class C prescription balance
   d) bulk prescription balance

14) What type of measuring device should be used to measure 3ml of a liquid for compounding?
   a) 5ml beaker
   b) 10ml conical graduate
   c) 2ml pipette
   d) 10ml cylindrical graduate

15) Grinding of tablets into a fine powder in a porcelain mortar is an example of;
   a) levigation
   b) trituration
   c) flocculation
   d) emulsification

16) Amoxicillin oral suspension is stable in a refrigerator for how many days after reconstitution?
   a) 7 days
   b) 10 days
   c) 14 days
   d) 20 days

17) Normal Saline (N.S.) contains;
   a) 0.45% NaCl
   b) 0.33% NaCl
   c) 9.0% NaCl
   d) 0.9% NaCl

18) Digoxin belongs to which drug classification?
   a) antiarrhythmic
   b) cardiac glycoside
   c) beta blocker
   d) Ca channel blocker

19) Which of the following drugs is a benzodiazepine?
    a) Fiorinal
    b) Percodan
    c) Demerol
    d) Klonopin

20) Which drug is most likely to cause a photosensitivity reaction?
    a) Biaxin
    b) penicillin VK
    c) Cipro
    d) tetracycline

21) What drug in a dose of 20mg qd, is used to treat dyspepsia?
    a) Lasix
    b) Pepcid
    c) Inderal
    d) Dilantin

22) The directions for use for Timoptic is ii gtts os bid.
    What is the meaning of os?
    a) both eyes
    b) right eye
    c) left eye
    d) left ear

23) What is the Latin abbreviation for "after meals"?
    a) ac
    b) pc
    c) qd
    d) hs

24) An order reads "Tylenol 325mg PR q4h prn." What dosage form
    should be
    dispensed?
    a) tablets
    b) capsules
    c) syrup
    d) suppositories

25) When repacking drugs, what expiration date will appear on the package?
    a) 3 months
    b) 6 months
    c) 50% of labeled expiration date to a maximum of 1 year
    d) the original expiration date on the bulk solid

26) The abbreviation "PCN" means what?
   a) allergy
   b) penicillin
   c) nothing by mouth
   d) carcinoma

27) Which drug is used as a "RESCUE" from toxicity of methotrexate?
   a) Ipecac
   b) Taxol injection
   c) leucovorin
   d) acetylcysteine

28) A patient hands you an empty vial of Ritalin and asks for the Rx to be refilled. What should you do?
   a) refill the Rx if the physician specified a refill
   b) ask the pharmacist to call the physician for a refill
   c) tell the patient that the medication is not refillable
   d) refill the Rx immediately

29) What is the proper procedure for cleaning a laminar flow hood?
   a) clean the hood from side to side starting from the front of the hood working towards the rear of the hood
   b) clean the plexiglass side with isopropyl alcohol
   c) wipe the hood with a damp cloth
   d) clean the hood from side to side starting from the back of the hood towards the front of the hood

30) Which procedure would you not do when opening an ampule?
   a) wipe the neck with an alcohol pad
   b) after wiping with an alcohol pad, dry the neck with a paper towel
   c) break the ampule with an alcohol pad covering the neck
   d) filter the contents with a filter needle upon withdrawal

31) How far within a hood should the pharmacy technician work?
   a) as far into the hood as possible
   b) 3 inches within the hood
   c) at least 6 inches within the hood
   d) anywhere within the hood is acceptable

32) What size filter is considered a sterilizing filter?
   a) 0.22 micron
   b) 0.3 micron
   c) 0.45 micron
   d) 5 micron

33) How often must a laminar flow hood be checked?
    a) every 3 months
    b) every 6 months
    c) once yearly
    d) when it breaks down

34) Which of the following drugs is not an OTC product?
    a) Poly-Vi-Sol drops
    b) Poly-Vi-Sol tablets
    c) Theragran-M tablets
    d) Poly-Vi-Flor drops

35) Which of the following drugs is not an OTC product?
    a) Advil
    b) Nuprin
    c) Ibuprofen 400mg tabs
    d) Tylenol suppositories

36) How long may a schedule II drug be refilled?
    a) 1 year
    b) 6 months or 5 refills
    c) no refills
    d) as many refills as the physician indicates

37) If a prescription states "refill prn," for how long may this Rx be refilled?
    a) 1 year
    b) 2 years
    c) 6 months
    d) until the patient has a new prescription filled

38) Which of the following drugs is a coronary vasodilator?
    a) meperidine
    b) diltiazem
    c) nitroglycerin
    d) piroxicam

39) What ratio of 25% dextrose and 10% dextrose should be mixed to make
     a 20% dextrose solution?
    a) 1:1
    b) 2:1
    c) 3:1
    d) 4:1

40) How many 100mg tablets will be needed to make 1/2 liter of a 1:250 solution?
   a) 10 tablets
   b) 15 tablets
   c) 20 tablets
   d) 30 tablets

41) Codeine, meperidine and oxycodone all belong to which controlled schedule?
   a) Schedule I
   b) Schedule II
   c) Schedule III
   d) Schedule IV

42) A physician prescribes Ceclor 375mg po bid. What is wrong with this prescription?
   a) the Rx lacks a drug strength
   b) the Rx lacks directions for use
   c) the Rx lacks a route of drug administration
   d) the Rx lacks a duration of therapy

43) How often must controlled substances be physically inventoried?
   a) once yearly
   b) once every 2 years
   c) twice yearly
   d) once every 3 years

44) Which of the following 2 drug classes have cross sensitivity?
   a) tetracycline and penicillin
   b) penicillin and erythromycin
   c) erythromycin and penicillin
   d) penicillin and cephalosporin

45) Which governmental agency is responsible for safety in the workplace?
   a) DEA
   b) NDA
   c) OSHA
   d) FDA

46) Which dosage form is formulated to dissolve in the intestine rather than the stomach?
   a) sublingual
   b) transdermal
   c) enteric-coated
   d) intranasal

47) Determine the flow rate of an IVPB containing 120ml of gentamicin, if the solution is to be infused over a 1 hour period and the administration set is calibrated to deliver 10 drops per ml.
a) 10 gtts/min
b) 20 gtts/min
c) 30 gtts/min
d) 40 gtts/min

48) A piggyback has 50ml of antibiotic infusing at a rate of 30 gtts/min. How long will it take for this solution to be administered if the set is calibrated to deliver 15 gtts/ml?
a) 15 minutes
b) 20 minutes
c) 25 minutes
d) 30 minutes

49) How many 10 mg minoxidil tablets would be needed to make 60 ml of a 2% solution?
a) 120 tablets
b) 60 tablets
c) 30 tablets
d) 10 tablets

50) Which nongovernmental agency is responsible for the accreditation of institutional settings?
a) AMA
b) ASHP
c) JCAHO
d) APhA

51) The process whereby a drug crosses a membrane into the blood stream is called:
a) absorption
b) distribution
c) metabolism
d) elimination

52) Which solution is recommended for cleaning a laminar flow hood?
a) soap and warm water
b) isopropyl alcohol
c) povidone-iodine
d) hydrogen peroxide

53) If a manufacturer's labeling results in a temporary adverse health consequence, what type of FDA recall would be instituted?
   a) Class I
   b) Class II
   c) Class III
   d) Class IV

54) Which of the following is an unacceptable DEA #?
   a) AH 2361424
   b) AH 1462136
   c) AH 3126426
   d) AH 1327142

55) A compounded prescription requires using 12 capsules costing $30.00 per 50 capsules and 120gm of an ointment base costing $7.50 per pound. If a $5.00 dispensing fee is included, how much should the patient be charged?
   a) $12.50
   b) $19.95
   c) $16.60
   d) $14.18

56) At which temperature should procaine penicillin G be stored?
   a) 2 - 8 degrees Centigrade
   b) 8 - 15 degrees Centigrade
   c) 15 - 30 degrees Centigrade
   d) 30 - 40 degrees Centigrade

57) What is the definition of "controlled room temperature?"
   a) 2 - 8 degrees Centigrade
   b) 8 - 15 degrees Centigrade
   c) 15 - 30 degrees Centigrade
   d) 30 - 40 degrees Centigrade

58) Which characteristic is not important when preparing an IV admixture?
   a) sterility
   b) palpability
   c) solubility
   d) stability

59) Which drug information source would the pharmacy technician check for a possible drug interaction?
   a) Redbook
   b) American Drug Index
   c) Remington's Pharmaceutical Sciences
   d) Facts and Comparisons

60) Insulin is to be added to an IV admixture. What type of insulin may be used?
   a) Regular
   b) Lente
   c) Ultra Lente
   d) Isophane

61) The process whereby a drug is transformed by the liver is called:
   a) absorption
   b) distribution
   c) metabolism
   d) elimination

62) What is "Syrup of Ipecac" indicated for?
   a) to suppress a dry cough
   b) to induce vomiting
   c) to relieve the itching from hives
   d) as a sweetening agent in pharmaceutical products

63) A patient enters the pharmacy complaining of persistent heartburn. The pharmacy technician should;
   a) tell the patient to call their physician
   b) tell the patient to go to the ER immediately
   c) tell the patient to speak to the pharmacist
   d) suggest the use of Tagamet HB

64) Which of the following duties may a pharmacy technician not do?
   a) enter prescription data into the computer
   b) call the wholesaler for a drug order
   c) affix a drug label to a prescription container
   d) accept a verbal medication order from a physician

65) Who implements formulary review?
   a) FDA
   b) P+T Committee
   c) OSHA
   d) JCAHO

66) Amoxicillin suspension requires which auxiliary label?
   a) Shake Well
   b) Shake Well and Refrigerate
   c) Shake Well and Drug May Discolor Urine
   d) Shake Well and Avoid Dairy Products

67) Cleocin suspension is available in a concentration of 75mg/5ml.
   How many ml are required for a 300mg dose?
   a) 10ml
   b) 15ml
   c) 20ml
   d) 25ml

68) Tagamet IV has been ordered to run at 2.5 drops/min. It contains 875mg of
   Tagamet in a total of 250ml. How many milligrams of Tagamet will the
   patient receive per hour if the set is calibrated to deliver 15 gtts/ml?
   a) 25mg/hr
   b) 30mg/hr
   c) 35mg/hr
   d) 40mg/hr

69) Another pharmacy calls for a copy of an Rx and the pharmacist is busy
   counselling a patient. The pharmacy technician should;
   a) convey the prescription information to the pharmacy
   b) interrupt the pharmacist
   c) ask the pharmacy to call the prescribing physician
   d) tell them that the pharmacist is busy and to call back later

70) Digoxin is available in a concentration of 0.1mg/ml. How many ml are
   required to administer a 75mcg dose?
   a) 1.0ml
   b) 0.75ml
   c) 0.5ml
   d) 0.25ml

71) Heparin is available in a vial labeled 20,000U/ml. How many ml are
   required for a 12,500U dose?
   a) 0.625ml
   b) 0.75ml
   c) 0.5ml
   d) 0.25ml

72) Mylanta and Donnatal are to be combined in a 2:1 ratio. How much of each is required to make 90ml of the suspension?
a) 75ml/15ml
b) 15ml/75ml
c) 60ml/30ml
d) 30ml/60ml

73) The directions for use of a medication are "ii gtts au q4h x5d."
The proper interpretation of "au" is:
a) in both eyes
b) in both ears
c) in right eye
d) in right ear

74) What is the proper method of measuring a liquid in a graduated cylinder?
a) hold at eye level and read the top of the meniscus
b) hold at eye level and read the bottom of the meniscus
c) place graduate on table and read meniscus from above
d) place graduate on table and read meniscus from below

75) The purpose of OSHA is to;
a) ensure safe and effective drug therapy
b) assign drug recall classifications
c) monitor OTC labeling requirements
d) assure a safe workplace

76) According to federal law, controlled substances must be safeguarded by all of the following EXCEPT;
a) dispensing records
b) storage records
c) transport records
d) inventory records

77) The process of producing a smooth dispersion of a drug with a spatula is called:
a) levigation
b) trituration
c) micturition
d) flocculation

78) Which of the following groups is usually not a member of the P+T Committee?
   a) medical representative
   b) nursing representative
   c) dental representative
   d) pharmacy representative

79) The purpose of the P+T Committee is to:
   a) establish and maintain a drug formulary system
   b) recommend policies regarding investigational drugs
   c) collect data from drug utilization review
   d) all the above

80) Which of the following drugs is not a beta blocking agent?
   a) Normodyne
   b) Lotensin
   c) Tenormin
   d) Lopressor

81) The AWP for a gallon (3785ml) of antihistamine/antitussive cough syrup is
   $18.75, with an additional 20% discount from the wholesaler.
   What is the cost of 1 pint of the medication?
   a) $3.25
   b) $2.75
   c) $1.40
   d) $1.87

82) The "C" designation for controlled substances must appear on a
   controlled prescription:
   a) in red in the lower left hand corner of the Rx
   b) in any color in the lower left hand corner of the Rx
   c) in red in the lower right hand corner of the Rx
   d) in any color in the lower right hand corner of the Rx

83) The device that links computers via communication lines is referred to
   as:
   a) transfer program
   b) modem
   c) disc drive
   d) RAM

84) A MSDS provides what type of product information?
   a) information concerning the side effects of the product
   b) information relating to the contraindications of the product
   c) information describing clinical trials of the product
   d) information regarding product ingredients

85) The directions on a prescription for prednisone 5 mg tablets reads:
Sig: 2 tabs po bid for 3 days, 3 tabs po qd for 2 days, 2 tabs po qd for 2 days,
1 tab po qd for 1 day then 1/2 tab po qd for 1 day. How many tablets should
be dispensed?
a) 22 tablets
b) 24 tablets
c) 26 tablets
d) 28 tablets

86) A vial of reconstituted Adriamycin breaks inside a vertical flow hood.
What should the technician do?
a) wipe up the spill with absorbent paper towels
b) dilute the spill with isopropyl alcohol
c) clean up the spill with a "spill kit"
d) dilute the spill with water

87) The Roman numerals XLII is equivalent to:
a) 42
b) 62
c) 402
d) 92

88) The pharmacy technician is asked to assist in the compounding of a
lotion. In what drug information source would this information be looked up?
a) PDR
b) Merck Manual
c) Facts and Comparisons
d) Remington's Pharmaceutical Sciences

89) If a pharmacy technician discovers a medication has expired, he/she should:
a) dispense the drug if it expired within the last week
b) discard the drug
c) follow the manufacturers return policy
d) dispense the drug at a discount price

90) What protective apparel must be worn when reconstituting a
chemotherapeutic agent?
a) 2 pair of gloves
b) a gown
c) a mask
d) all the above

91) 1+1/2 tablespoonsful is equivalent to how many ml?
   a) 7.5ml
   b) 22.5ml
   c) 17.5ml
   d) 12.5ml

92) How many ounces are contained in one pint?
   a) 8
   b) 12
   c) 16
   d) 18

93) Which of the following drugs requires the auxiliary label
   "May Discolor Urine Red"?
   a) Bactrim DS
   b) Vibramycin
   c) Cipro
   d) Pyridium

94) Which federal legislation enacted in 1970 regulates the use and
   distribution of substances with high abuse potential?
   a) FDCA
   b) CSA
   c) DEA
   d) FDA

95) Which of the following drugs is not a laxative?
   a) Dulcolax
   b) Metamucil
   c) Imodium
   d) Colace

96) U-100 insulin contains:
   a) 100 units per 10 ml
   b) 100 units per 1 ml
   c) 100 units per 1/2 ml
   d) none of the above

97) A formula for a cough syrup contains 1 gr of codeine per fluid ounce. How
many grains are contained in one teaspoonful?
   a) 1/2 gr
   b) 1/4 gr
   c) 1/6 gr
   d) 1/8 gr

98) How many mls of water should be added to 95% ethyl alcohol to make one liter of a 30% ethyl alcohol solution?
a) 685 ml
b) 315 ml
c) 750 ml
d) 250 ml

99) A patient on warfarin therapy should never take which of the following medications?
a) Percocet
b) Tylenol
c) Demerol
d) Percodan

100) Which of the following is a Schedule IV controlled substance?
a) Lomotil
b) Xanax
c) Demerol
d) Haldol

101) The pharmacy technician receives a call from a patient that indicates their 16 month old child has just ingested half a bottle of Children's Tylenol. What may the pharmacy technician _not_ do?
a) ask them to speak to the pharmacist
b) tell them to induce vomiting immediately
c) give them the number to the poison control center
d) tell them to go to the nearest ER

102) If 15 grams of hydrocortisone 1% ointment are combined with 30 grams of a hydrocortisone 2.5% ointment, what is the percentage of hydrocortisone in the final product?
a) 1.25%
b) 1.5%
c) 1.75%
d) 2.0%

103) What volume of 24% trichloroacetic acid (TCA) is needed to prepare eight 3 ounce bottles of 10% TCA solution?
a) 100ml
b) 200ml
c) 300ml
d) 400ml

144

104) Nitrostat 1/200gr is equivalent to how many milligrams?
a) 0.6mg
b) 0.5mg
c) 0.4mg
d) 0.3mg

105) After reconstitution, how should the drug filgrastim be stored?
a) at room temperature for 24 hours
b) in the refrigerator or at room temp for 7 days
c) in the freezer
d) there are no specific storage requirements for this drug

106) How many gallons are contained in 144 pints?
a) 17
b) 18
c) 19
d) 20

107) 185ml is equivalent to how many fluid ounces?
a) 5.75
b) 6.0
c) 6.17
d) 6.5

108) Heparin belongs to which pharmacological category?
a) anticonvulsant
b) anticoagulant
c) antibiotic
d) antipsychotic

109) When a drug is filtered by the kidney into the bladder, this process is called:
a) absorption
b) secretion
c) distribution
d) elimination

110) The computer program used for dispensing medication in the pharmacy setting is referred to as:
a) hardware
b) mediumware
c) software
d) modem

111) Goals, Policies and Procedures, and Mission Statements are all examples of:
a) strategic planning
b) tactical planning
c) emergency planning
d) risk management

112) Which of the following drugs is an antiarrhythmic?
a) Panadol
b) Pravachol
c) Prolixin
d) Pronestyl

113) The dispensing label on an outpatient pharmacy prescription requires:
a) manufacturers lot #
b) physicians DEA #
c) legal name of pharmacy and address
d) physicians state license #

114) A TPN order is to contain 2mg/l of folic acid. If the stock vial of folic acid contains 5mg/ml, what volume would be required to prepare 3000ml of TPN?
a) 0.6 ml
b) 0.8 ml
c) 1.0 ml
d) 1.2 ml

115) Efudex cream:
a) may be used as an anti-infective
b) should be applied 3-4 times daily
c) should be applied with gloves or a nonmetallic object
d) is available as an OTC product

116) Therapeutic equivalency indicates that the two drugs:
a) are the same shape and color
b) have the same quantity of active ingredient
c) belong to the same therapeutic class
d) are equally effective at the same dose

117) Materials management refers to:
a) the drug procurement process
b) inventory control
c) drug storage
d) all the above

118) The red "C" in the lower right corner of a prescription designates
     that the drug is:
     a) Schedule I controlled substance only
     b) Schedule II controlled substance only
     c) Schedule II, III, IV or V controlled substances
     d) all the above

119) When developing a policy and procedure for ensuring the safety of a
     drug in a multidose vial, all the following should be considered except:
     a) the cost of the medication
     b) the stability of the medication
     c) the presence of a suitable preservative
     d) all the above

120) Scanning for drug prices and stock levels would be accomplished with
     which device?
     a) compiler
     b) modem
     c) barcode reader
     d) zip-drive

121) An "automatic stop order" in the institutional setting would apply to which
     category of drugs?
     a) antidepressants
     b) antipsychotics
     c) antibiotics
     d) antihypertensives

122) The initial dose of aminophylline for a nonsmoking adult is 0.7mg/kg/hr for
     12 hours. How many ml of an IV solution containing 400mg per 100ml would
     be required for a 154lb male over a 12 hour period?
     a) 127ml
     b) 147ml
     c) 167ml
     d) 187ml

123) The pharmacy technician is asked to divide 5 liters of Nilstat suspension
     into an equal number of 10ml and 15ml unit dose dispensing cups. How many
     10 ml dispensing cups can be made from this quantity of suspension?
     a) 200
     b) 250
     c) 333
     d) 500

124) The appearance of crystals in mannitol injecton indicates:
   a) that the solution contains impurities and should be discarded
   b) that the solution is outdated
   c) that the solution may be unstable and should be returned for credit
   d) that the solution is cold and the crystals may be redissolved

125) Which of the following medications is an anticonvulsant?
   a) atenolol
   b) dextromethorphan
   c) carbamazepine
   d) isoxsuprine

ANSWERS TO PRACTICE TEST #1

SEE NEXT PAGE

ANSWER KEY FOR PRACTICE TEST #1

1) b	26) b	51) a	76) c	101) b
2) d	27) c	52) b	77) a	102) d
3) a	28) c	53) b	78) c	103) c
4) c	29) d	54) c	79) d	104) d
5) c	30) b	55) d	80) b	105) b
6) d	31) c	56) a	81) d	106) b
7) b	32) a	57) c	82) c	107) c
8) a	33) b	58) b	83) b	108) b
9) d	34) d	59) d	84) d	109) d
10) b	35) c	60) a	85) b	110) c
11) a	36) c	61) c	86) c	111) a
12) b	37) a	62) b	87) a	112) d
13) a	38) c	63) c	88) d	113) c
14) d	39) b	64) d	89) c	114) d
15) b	40) c	65) b	90) d	115) c
16) c	41) b	66) b	91) b	116) b
17) d	42) d	67) c	92) c	117) d
18) b	43) b	68) c	93) d	118) c
19) d	44) d	69) d	94) b	119) a
20) d	45) c	70) b	95) c	120) c
21) b	46) c	71) a	96) b	121) c
22) c	47) b	72) c	97) c	122) b
23) b	48) c	73) b	98) a	123) a
24) d	49) a	74) b	99) d	124) d
25) c	50) c	75) d	100) b	125) c

PRACTICE EXAM # 2

1) Which of the following drugs is a NSAID?
   a) Toradol
   b) Bretylol
   c) Efficol
   d) Geritol

2) Tagamet, Axid, and Pepcid are examples of :
   a) dopamine receptor blockers
   b) H2 receptor blockers
   c) ACE Inhibitors
   d) beta blockers

3) What is the % equivalent of a 1 : 8 ratio ?
   a) 12.5%
   b) 14.5%
   c) 16.5%
   d) 18.5%

4) What would be the proper course of action if a technician accidentally
   had skin contact with a cytotoxic drug?
   a) call 911
   b) wash hands thoroughly with soap and water immediately
   c) wash hands thoroughly with soap and water immediately and seek
      medical attention
   d) read the P+P Manual and follow stated instructions

5) How would you identify a medication in a drug recall situation?
   a) by its generic name
   b) by its trade name
    c) by the manufacturers bar code
   d) by the drugs lot #

6) Which of the following is the most accurate device for measuring liquids?
   a) cylindrical graduate
   b) conical graduate
   c) beaker
   d) a 2oz. cup

7) Narcan is categorized as a :
    a) narcotic agonist
    b) dopamine agonist
    c) narcotic antagonist
    d) dopamine antagonist

8) Which of the following medications is commercially available as a patch?
    a) morphine
    b) meperidine
    c) codeine
    d) fentanyl

9) Which of the following is an example of a side effect of antineoplastic
    therapy?
    a) bone marrow suppression
    b) increased red blood cell formation
    c) increased white blood cell formation
    d) increased platelet formation

10) The NDC on a medication bottle refers to the:
    a) manufacturer
    b) drug product
    c) quantity packaged
    d) all the above

11) How old must a person be to sign the exempt narcotic log:
    a) 16 years old
    b) 18 years old
    c) 21 years old
    d) 25 years old

12) Which of the following dosage forms is formulated to mask an objectionable
    taste of a medication?
    a) sublingual tablets
    b) chewable tablets
    c) buccal tablets
    d) film-coated tablets

13) Which of the following dosage forms has the highest concentration of
    alcohol in its formulation?
    a) a syrup
    b) an elixir
    c) a tincture
    d) an emulsion

14) The dose of cefaclor in children is 20mg/kg/day in divided doses.
    A prescription for an 82 lb youngster prescribes 375mg PO TID. After bringing
    this prescription to the attention of the pharmacist, the pharmacist agrees that
    there is a problem with this prescription. The problem is:
    a) the dose prescribed is subtherapeutic
    b) the dose prescribed is an overdose
    c) the drug is not available in this strength
    d) tell the patient to break a 750mg into two equal parts

15) A hermetically sealed container is impervious to:
    a) radiation
    b) sunlight
    c) air
    d) none of the above

16) Which of the following medications is an OTC analgesic?
    a) FeSO4 tablets
    b) diphenhydramine capsules
    c) ketoprofen tablets
    d) DSS capsules

17) What is the maximum number of refills permitted for a Schedule III
    medication?
    a) 5 refills
    b) no refills
    c) 1 refill
    d) prn refills

18) Amphotericin B is available in a concentration of 50mg/10ml. What quantity
    is required for a 3mg test dose?
    a) 0.1ml
    b) 0.2ml
    c) 0.3ml
    d) 0.6ml

19) Patient information for Cerumenex would include the following:
    a) how to instill eye drops
    b) how to apply and rotate a patch medication
    c) how to instill ear drops
    d) how to use an inhaler properly

152

20) How many units of NPH U-100 would be administered if the patient's noon dose was 0. 25ml?
   a) 15 units
   b) 30 units
   c) 25 units
   d) 50 units

21) Who is responsible for the drug recall process?
   a) OSHA
   b) OBRA
   c) FDA
   d) NBA

22) Oral syringes are:
   a) available in two sizes
   b) sterile products
   c) made from glass only
   d) unable to accept a luer-lock needle

23) Which of the following is NOT a technician responsibility?
   a) signing the DEA form from the wholesaler
   b) assisting in the controlled substance inventory
   c) prepacking of controlled substances
   d) preparing controlled substance dispensing report

24) A patient weighing 110 lbs is to receive 5mcg/kg/min of a IV solution containing Dopamine 600mg in 250ml D5W. The calculated IV dose rate is:
   a) 125mcg/min
   b) 0.125mg/min
   c) 0.250mg/min
   d) 25mcg/min

25) A homecare pharmacy compounds 50 TPN orders daily. Which device would assist in the preparation of these orders?
   a) Baxter ATM machine
   b) Automix
   c) Macromix
   d) Automated System Mixer

26) What is the storage requirement for reconstituted cefaclor 250mg/5ml?
   a) -4 to 14 degrees F
   b) 36 to 46 degrees F
   c) 46 to 59 degrees F
   d) 59 to 86 degrees F

27) Which of the following medications is availble by prescription only?
      a) phenylephrine
      b) loperamide
      c) diphenhydramine
      d) phenytoin

28) Which of the following statements is appropriate for a laminar flow hood?
      a) test the HEPA filter every 2 years
      b) work at least 3 inches within the hood
      c) clean the hood from back to front
      d) clean the hood from front to back

29) Needles used to prepare IV solutions should be discarded by;
      a) snipping them into a Sharp's Container
      b) ziplocking them in bags labeled " Biohazardous Waste "
      c) throwing them away with the regular trash
      d) placing them in a recycle bin for sterilization

30) The markup for a $36.75 vial of antibiotic is 18%. What is the retail price for this
      medication?
      a) $39.67
      b) $41.68
      c) $43.36
      d) $46.92

31) Which of the following products would be contraindicated in a patient who
      has had an anaphylactic reaction to ASA?
      a) Percocet
      b) Percodan
      c) Tylox
      d) Fioricet/codeine

32) What is the therapeutic generic equivalent for Benadryl?
      a) ephedrine
      b) phenylpropanolamine
      c) phenylephrine
      d) diphenhydramine

33) Which of the following auxiliary labels should be affixed to a prescription for
      diphenhydramine elixir?
      a) May Discolor Urine
      b) May Cause Drowsiness
      c) Take With Food or Milk
      d) Shake Well and Refrigerate

34) What is the resultant percentage concentration when 30gms of codeine phosphate is dissolved in 2 liters of solution?
   a) 1.0%
   b) 10%
   c) 1.5%
   d) 15%

35) Schedule II medications must be ordered in which of the following ways?
   a) completing the proper DEA form
   b) calling the manufacturer directly
   c) calling the wholesaler directly
   d) calling the Bureau of Controlled Substances

36) Which of the following routes of administration produces the quickest onset \ of action of a drug?
   a) PR
   b) PO
   c) IM
   d) IV

37) Which auxiliary label should be affixed to the vial when dispensing metronidazole?
   a) May Discolor Urine
   b) May Cause Drowsiness
   c) Shake Well and Refrigerate
   d) Do Not Drink Alcoholic Beverages

38) The directions for Fosamax states "10mg po qd pc." The technician should bring this to the pharmacist's attention because:
   a) the medication is not available in a 10 mg dose
   b) the medication should be taken 1/2 hour before breakfast
   c) the normal dose is 10mg TID
   d) the medication may be taken before or after meals

39) Which of the following is NOT required on a unit-dosed packaged drug?
   a) expiration date
   b) lot #
   c) storage requirements
   d) strength of medication

40) A 500 tablet bottle of ferrous sulfate costs $17.86. What would be the cost of 39 tablets?
    a) $1.78
    b) $1.39
    c) $ 2.87
    d) $2.43

41) An overdose of morphine would cause:
    a) diarrhea
    b) enlarged pupils
    c) CNS stimulation
    d) respiratory depression

42) Which of the following medications would be used to treat an ear infection?
    a) SMZ-TMP
    b) AZT
    c) INH
    d) HCTZ

43) If a patient cannot tolerate a NSAID, which one of the following medications may he/she take?
    a) indomethacin
    b) piroxicam
    c) acetaminophen
    d) ketorolac

44) A Patient Package Insert must be dispensed with which of the following medications?
    a) norethindrone
    b) betamethasone
    c) spironolactone
    d) prednisone

45) What volume of pediatric digoxin injection 0.1mg/ml is required for a 50mcg dose?
    a) 0.5ml
    b) 0.75ml
    c) 1.5ml
    d) 1.75ml

156

46) A prescription states "Norvasc 5mg #100 1 tab po qd." If the third party coverage limits the dispensing to a 30 day supply, the pharmacy should:
    a) dispense a 30 day supply with no refills
    b) dispense a 100 day supply and have the patient pay the difference
    c) call the third party payor and get special permission to dispense 100
    d) dispense a 30 day supply with refills

47) A third party insurance program pays for only a 14 day supply of a specific medication. If the directions for use read " i - ii tabs po q3-4h prn," what is the maximum allowable quantity to be dispensed?
    a) 84 tablets
    b) 112 tablets
    c) 168 tablets
    d) 224 tablets

48) How much of 90% ethanol must be mixed with 10% ethanol to make 1 pint of a 40% ethanol solution?
    a) 161ml of 90% + 312ml of 10%
    b) 177ml of 90% + 296ml of 10%
    c) 196ml of 90% + 277ml of 10%
    d) 207ml of 90% + 266ml of 10%

49) The primary function of the P+T Committee is to:
    a) set standards for credentialing of the pharmacy staff
    b) work with the State Board of Pharmacy to enforce pharmacy standards
    c) establish standards for therapeutics
    d) act as a liaison between medical and pharmacy staffs

50) Federal law requires which of the following information to be documented on a daily basis?
    a) a log of controlled substances dispensed
    b) patient profiles of prescriptions dispensed for the first time
    c) a running inventory of all drugs dispensed
    d) incident reports on mislabeled drugs

51) Federal regulations require a Package Patient Insert (PPI) to be dispensed each time when which medication is dispensed?
    a) nitroglycerin patches
    b) antibiotic eye drops
    c) analgesics containing codeine derivatives
    d) estrogens

52) Which of the following medications belongs to the same class of drugs as etodolac?
   a) phenylephrine
   b) diclofenac
   c) haloperidol
   d) cefaclor

53) The Patient Package Insert (PPI) for oral contraceptives is required to be dispensed:
   a) each time the prescription is dispensed
   b) only upon the request of the prescriber
   c) the first time the prescription is dispensed
   d) is never dispensed with the prescription

54) A prescription reads " hydrocortisone 1%, clotrimazole 1%, aa ap qhs".
   How many gms of hydrocortisone would be required to make 90gms?
   a) 30gms HC + 60gms clotrimazole
   b) 60gms HC + 30gms clotrimazole
   c) 45gms HC + 45gms clotrimazole
   d) 15gms HC + 75gms clotrimazole

55) The Poison Prevention Packaging Act requires childproof packaging for all medications except:
   a) prednisone
   b) nitroglycerin
   c) isosorbide dinitrate sl
   d) ASA 5gr

56) Which of the following medicatons is a Schedule IV controlled substance?
   a) paregoric
   b) triazolam
   c) diphenoxylate with atropine
   d) dronabinol

57) How much Ceclor 250mg/5ml suspension should be dispensed for a 375mg dose?
   a) 0.75ml
   b) 1.25ml
   c) 7.5ml
   d) 12.5ml

58) To which drug classification does the drug prochlorperazine belong?
    a) antifungal
    b) antibiotic
    c) antiemetic
    d) antineoplastic

59) The computer term " mneumonic" is defined as:
    a) a shortened term used to facilitate data entry
    b) a barcode used for reordering medications
    c) a special font used for pharmacy symbols
    d) a back-up hard drive to store prescription information

60) What type of Drug Recall occurs when a drug is not likely to cause a temporary adverse health consequence?
    a) no recall is required
    b) Class III recall
    c) Class II recall
    d) Class I recall

61) A retail pharmacy receives an extra 1/2% discount on a $437.89 invoice from the wholesaler. This calculates to be a savings of:
    a) $218.95
    b) $21.90
    c) $2.19
    d) $0.22

62) Which of the following federal regulations requires that a pharmacist counsel Medicaid patients?
    a) Medication Safety Act
    b) Omnibus Budget Reconciliation Act
    c) Health and Safety Act
    d) Patient Counseling Act

63) What information is required to be posted on each cell of an automated counting device?
    a) name, strength and NDC code of drug
    b) name, strength and DEA # of the drug
    c) name, strength, lot# and expiration date of drug
    d) name, strength and date cell was filled

64) Phenytoin is available in which dosage form?
   a) 200mg sustained-release capsules
   b) 100mg chewable tablets
   c) 125mg/5ml oral solution
   d) 30mg/5ml oral solution

65) What volume of Betadine Solution would be needed to prepackage
   152 pints?
   a) 38 gallons
   b) 19 gallons
   c) 9.5 gallons
   d) 4.75 gallons

66) The term " AWP " stands for :
   a) American Way Products
   b) Automated Wholesaler Pricing
   c) Automation With Perfection
   d) Average Wholesale Price

67) Digoxin Elixir is available in a concentration of 0.05mg/ml. What quantity is
   required for a 0.125mg dose?
   a) 2.0 ml
   b) 2.5 ml
   c) 3.0 ml
   d) 3.5 ml

68) Which category of drugs stimulates the release of insulin in the body?
   a) hypoglycemic agents
   b) hyperglycemic agents
   c) hypoallergenic agents
   d) hyperallergenic agents

69) Terbutaline belongs to which drug classification?
   a) antineoplastic
   b) antiflatulent
   c) bronchodilator
   d) antihypertensive

70) Which drug information source would a technician use for information
   concerning the dosing of a newly marketed antihypertensive?
   a) Remington's Pharmaceutical Sciences
   b) Facts and Comparisons
   c) USP - NF
   d) Clinical Toxicology of Commercial Products

160

71) If a third party payor specifies a maximum 1 month supply for a specific drug and the directions for use state " i cap po qid," how many units of the drug may be dispensed?
   a) 124
   b) 112
   c) 180
   d) 120

72) Which problem can be avoided by administering a drug IV?
   a) local irritation
   b) infiltration
   c) aspiration
   d) intoxication

73) Which of the following medications is cause for concern in patients allergic to ASA?
   a) bismuth subsalicylate
   b) lovastatin
   c) meclizine
   d) vitamin A

74) Which class of drugs would be administered for a dry, hacking cough?
   a) antitussive
   b) expectorant
   c) nasal decongestant
   d) antibiotic

75) Penicillin V is commercially available in which strength?
   a) 1.2 million units
   b) 400mg
   c) 2.4 million units
   d) 500mg

76) The " C " designation for controlled substances applies to:
   a) Schedule II drugs
   b) Schedule I + II drugs
   c) Schedule I - IV
   d) Schedule I - V

77) Tetracycline should not be administered with which of the following beverages?
   a) apple juice
   b) orange juice
   c) milk
   d) water

78) Consider the following RX: Depakote 250mg #180
                                  SIG: 1 tab po tid refill x3
   How many tablets should be dispensed for a 30 day supply?
        a) 60 tablets
        b) 90 tablets
        c) 120 tablets
        d) 180 tablets

79) What quantity of dexamethasone 0.75mg tablets will be required
    for a 4.5mg dose?
        a) 2 tablets
        b) 4 tablets
        c) 6 tablets
        d) 8 tablets

80) Rx: Cefixime 100mg/5ml
            SIG: 60mg po qd x10

    What volume of medication would be required for a single daily dose?
        a)1.25 ml
        b) 2.0 ml
        c) 2.5 ml
        d) 3.0 ml

81) The CDC is the regulatory commission responsible for:
        a) infection control
        b) hazardous drugs
        c) new drug applications
        d) waste disposal

82) Which of the following vitamins are fat soluble?
        a) vitamins B and C
        b) vitamins A, D, E and K
        c) thiamine and riboflavin
        d) all the above

83) Methylphenidate belongs to which schedule of controlled substances?
        a) CI
        b) CII
        c) CIII
        d) CIV

84) NTG is prescribed for the treatment of:
    a) hypertension
    b) arrhythmias
    c) angina pectoris
    d) hyperglycemia

85) If a prescription is labeled " ii gtts au tid" , the drug product may be:
    a) Cortisporin Otic
    b) Cortisporin Ophthalmic
    c) Cortisporin Topical Cream
    d) any of the above products could be dispensed

86) What volume of a 125mg/ml injectable should be drawn up
    for a 175mg dose?
    a) 1.2 ml
    b) 1.4 ml
    c) 1.6 ml
    d) 1.8 ml

87) If state and federal pharmacy law differ, which law applies?
    a) local law
    b) state law
    c) federal law
    d) the more stringent law

88) Which of the following drugs is a calcium channel blocker?
    a) quinidine
    b) digoxin
    c) nifedipine
    d) captopril

89) The cost of 500 tablets of ibuprofen 400mg is $62.28. If your pharmacy
    marks up the cost by 13% and adds a $2.35 dispensing fee, what would
    be the retail charge for 120 tablets?
    a) $18.52
    b) $19.23
    c) $ 20.37
    d) $ 21.69

90) If a patient has a severe adverse reaction after prior administration of a drug, this would be referred to as:
   a) an anaphylactic reaction
   b) a drug misadventure
   c) a habituation reaction
   d) an antianxiety reaction

91) The purpose of a horizontal laminar flow hood is to:
   a) protect the technician when compounding sterile products
   b) sterilize the admixture
   c) provide a sterile environment for admixture compounding
   d) provide a clean surface for compounding sterile products

92) Lovastatin would be prescribed to:
   a) decrease blood pressure
   b) increase blood sugar
   c) treat a fungal infection
   d) decrease cholesterol

93) Reconstituted Ceclor is stable in the refrigerator for:
   a) 10 days
   b) 14 days
   c) 21 days
   d) 28 days

94) Needle gauge represents:
   a) the length of the needle
   b) the diameter of the needle
   c) the size of the hub of the needle
   d) none of the above

95) The AWP for a drug is $24.65 with a 17% discount from the wholesaler. What would be the net cost of this drug?
   a) $20.21
   b) $20.46
   c) $20.63
   d) $20.87

96) What is the total amount of hydrocortisone found in eight 1ounce tubes of hydrocortisone cream 2.5%?
   a) 6 gms
   b) 8 gms
   c) 10 gms
   d) 12 gms

97) Label directions for a prescription read " ii gtts os q4h x5d." Where should this medication be instilled?
    a) in the right eye
    b) in the right ear
    c) in the left eye
    d) in the left ear

98) The chemical structure for sodium bicarbonate is:
    a) $Na_2H_2CO_3$
    b) NaH_2CO_3
    c) $NaHCO_4$
    d) $NaHCO_3$

99) After syringes are used for preparation of hazardous substances, the pharmacy technician should:
    a) clip the needle and place it in the Sharp's Container
    b) recap the needle and place it in the Sharp's Container
    c) place the syringes in a sealed plastic bag and dispose in special waste
    d) any of the above would be proper disposal

100) All of the following preparations contain ibuprofen except:
    a) Advil
    b) Anacin
    c) Motrin
    d) Nuprin

101) What is the cost of 65 tablets if 120 tablets cost $8.73?
    a) $4.73
    b) $5.67
    c) $6.59
    d) $7.42

102) Who is responsible for the initial ordering of investigational drugs?
    a) P+T Committee
    b) nursing
    c) pharmacy
    d) MD

103) Which of the following medications is prescribed to treat CHF?
    a) carbamazepine
    b) doxycycline
    c) captopril
    d) glipizide

104) The purpose of complying with "Universal Precautions" is to:
    a) prevent the spread of communicable diseases
    b) prevent the transmission of blood-borne pathogens
    c) prevent contamination of sterile equipment
    d) all the above

105) If a Kg of an ointment contains 350gms of active ingredient, what is
    the percentage strength of the ointment?
    a) 25%
    b) 35%
    c) 50%
    d) 70%

106) DEA form 222 allows the pharmacy to:
    a) manufacture controlled substances
    b) order controlled substances
    c) destroy controlled substances
    d) all the above

107) Which of the following medications is available in transdermal form?
    a) codeine
    b) diazepam
    c) clonidine
    d) clonazepam

108) The first set of numbers of an NDC code identifies the:
    a) drug product
    b) dosage form
    c) package size
    d) manufacturer

109) What volume of digoxin 0.5mg/2ml injection will deliver a dose of 0.125mg?
    a) 1/4 ml
    b) 1/3 ml
    c) 1/8 ml
    d) 1/2 ml

110) Drugs within which class of Controlled Substances contain no legal use?
    a) C IV
    b) C III
    c) C II
    d) C I

111) How many mgs of diazepam are contained in 2.5ml of
    diazepam 10mg/2ml injection?
        a) 12 mgs
        b) 12.5mgs
        c) 15 mgs
        d) 17.5 mgs

112) The two-letter code assigned by the Orange Book indicates the:
        a) least expensive generic equivalent available
        b) bioavailability of generic drugs
        c) therapeutic equivalence of generic drugs
        d) none of the above

        a) access prescription files
        b) exit the program when finished
        c) transmit data off-line
        d) maintain prescription computer files

114) Which class of drugs decreases the viscosity of respiratory tract secretions?
        a) antihistamines
        b) vasoconstrictors
        c) antitussives
        d) expectorants

115) The pharmacist must complete DEA Form 222 to obtain which of the
    following medications?
        a) alprazolam
        b) acetaminophen with codeine
        c) oxycodone
        d) butabarbital

116) An abnormal irregular heartbeat is referred to as:
        a) bradycardia
        b) arrhythmia
        c) tachycardia
        d) fibrillation

117) Pharmacoeconomics refers to:
        a) drug expense and outcome data analysis
        b) the number of prescriptions filled
        c) the number of compounded prescriptions filled
        d) all of the above

118) The pharmacy technician is filling a prescription for Zithromax and
    notices in the patient profile that the patient is taking EES tablets.
    This is an example of:
    a) a drug interaction
    b) a contraindication
    c) a therapeutic duplication
    d) an adverse reaction

119) The active ingredient of a drug product is labeled USP. This standard
    is set forth in:
    a) the United States Pharmacy Act
    b) the United States Pharmacopeia
    c) the National Formulary
    d) the United States Pharmacy Service

120) Cocaine belongs to which category of controlled substances?
    a) C I
    b) C II
    c) C III
    d) C IV

121) Phenytoin is available in which dosage forms?
    a) tablets
    b) capsules
    c) IV injection
    d) all the above

122) If 75 gms of codeine phosphate is dissolved in 3 liters of sterile water,
    what is the resultant percentage strength of the solution?
    a) 0.25%
    b) 2.5%
    c) 25%
    d) 250%

123) The dose of cefamandole for children 3 months or older is 50-100mg/kg/day.
    What would be the daily dose range for a child who weighs 40 lbs?
    a) 2 - 4 gms per day
    b) 200 - 400 mgs per day
    c) 0.6 -1.2 gms per day
    d) 900 -1800 mgs per day

124) Which of the following ophthalmic medications must be refrigerated?
   a) Tobrex
   b) Gantrisin
   c) Genoptic
   d) Viroptic

125) The concentration of an injectable drug is 20mg/2.5ml. What volume
   would be required for an 8mg dose?
   a) 0.75 ml
   b) 1.0 ml
   c) 1.25 ml
   d) 1.5 ml

ANSWERS TO PRACTICE TEST #2

SEE NEXT PAGE

ANSWERS TO PRACTICE EXAM #2

1) a	26) b	51) d	76) d	101) a
2) b	27) d	52) b	77) c	102) d
3) a	28) c	53) a	78) b	103) c
4) c	29) a	54) c	79) c	104) b
5) d	30) c	55) b	80) d	105) b
6) a	31) b	56) b	81) a	106) b
7) c	32) d	57) c	82) b	107) c
8) d	33) b	58) c	83) b	108) d
9) a	34) c	59) a	84) c	109) d
10) d	35) a	60) b	85) a	110) d
11) b	36) d	61) c	86) b	111) b
12) d	37) d	62) b	87) d	112) c
13) c	38) b	63) c	88) c	113) a
14) b	39) c	64) c	89) b	114) d
15) c	40) b	65) b	90) a	115) c
16) c	41) d	66) d	91) c	116) b
17) a	42) a	67) b	92) d	117) d
18) d	43) c	68) a	93) b	118) c
19) c	44) a	69) c	94) b	119) b
20) c	45) a	70) b	95) b	120) a
21) c	46) d	71) d	96) a	121) d
22) d	47) d	72) c	97) c	122) b
23) a	48) b	73) a	98) d	123) d
24) c	49) c	74) a	99) c	124) d
25) b	50) a	75) d	100) b	125) b

PRACTICE EXAM #3

1) Which of the following medications is a Schedule IV Controlled Substance?
 a) Xanax
 b) Lomotil
 c) Tylox
 d) Tylenol #4

2) Which of the following Diagnostic Kits tests for glucose in the urine?
 a) Glucostix
 b) Chemstrip BG
 c) Clinistix
 d) Chemstrip K

3) What is the storage requirement for the drug Neupogen?
 a) room temperature
 b) cool temperature
 c) refrigerate
 d) freeze

4) The five schedules of controlled substances were established
 on the basis of:
 a) efficacy
 b) abuse potential
 c) medical use
 d) all of the above

5) Which of the following medications would be prescribed to treat
 a bacterial infection?
 a) acyclovir
 b) loperamide
 c) valproic acid
 d) metronidazole

6) The purchasing of drugs directly from the manufacturer requires:
 a) a minimum order set by the manufacturer
 b) that you dispense only their brand named medications
 c) that you do not purchase the drug from a wholesaler
 d) none of the above

7) To prepare sterile products, the laminar flow hood should be running for a minimum of:
   a) 15 minutes
   b) 30 minutes
   c) 45 minutes
   d) 60 minutes

8) A "Capital Expense" includes the following except:
   a) payroll
   b) shelving
   c) fixtures
   d) computer hardware

9) Federal law requires that all controlled substances dispensed bear the following statement on the dispensing label?
   a) Federal law prohibits the transfer of this drug to another person.
   b) This prescription may be habit forming.
   c) Federal law prohibits dispensing without a prescription.
   d) none of the above

10) Which of the following drugs is prescribed for the relief of allergy symptoms?
   a) pseudoephedrine
   b) phenylephrine
   c) antihistamines
   d) all the above

11) Needles used to prepare sterile IV solutions should be disposed in:
   a) biohazardous waste
   b) regular waste
   c) plastic bags
   d) Sharp's Container

12) The term "buccal" refers to the dosage form in which the drug is administered:
   a) sublingually
   b) in the buttocks
   c) in the cheek area
   d) behind the ear

13) A 3:1 TPN refers to:
    a) 3 parts lipid to one part dextrose
    b) lipids, dextrose and amino acids all in one bag
    c) 3 parts amino acid to one part lipid
    d) 3 days supply are contained in one bag

14) If a prescription is written for generic Anaprox DS, which medication should be dispensed?
    a) naproxen 220mg
    b) naproxen 440mg
    c) naproxen 500mg
    d) naproxen 550mg

15) Who is responsible for ordering investigational drugs?
    a) physician
    b) director of pharmacy services
    c) director of nursing
    d) only a Pharm. D

16) Which of the following drugs is a proton pump inhibitor?
    a) famotidine
    b) misoprostol
    c) lansoprazole
    d) ranitidine

17) If the pharmacy technician is to prepare 2 liters of a 6% Betadine Solution for stock, what volume of a 10% Betadine Solution would be used if it is mixed with distilled water?
    a) 600 ml
    b) 1200 ml
    c) 1500 ml

18) Generic Percodan contains:
    a) oxycodone and ASA
    b) oxycodone and APAP
    c) hydrocodone and ASA
    d) hydrocodone and APAP

19) If a drug product is acquired for $30 and sold for $35, what is the % markup?
    a) 8%
    b) 10%
    c) 12%
    d) 16%

20) The pharmacy refrigerator must be maintained at which of the following temperatures?
   a) 15 - 30 degrees F
   b) 36 - 46 degrees F
   c) 46-59 degrees F
   d) 59 - 86 degrees F

21) The diagnosis CHF refers to disease state involving which organ?
   a) liver
   b) kidney
   c) skin
   d) heart

22) What is the total weight if 0.05g is added to 500mcg?
   a) 50 mg
   b) 50.5mg
   c) 55mg
   D) 550mg

23) If amoxicillin 225mg po tid is ordered, how many mls of the 125mg/5ml suspension would be administered per dose?
   a) 7mls
   b) 8mls
   c) 9mls
   d) 10mls

24) What dosage forms are commercially available for the drug Flagyl?
   a) tablets only
   b) tablets and suspension
   c) tablets and IV
   d) tablets, suspension and IV

25) How many 250mg doses are contained in 5gms of Cephalexin?
   a) 5 doses
   b) 10 doses
   c) 15 doses
   d) 20 doses

26) Which auxiliary label should be affixed to a prescription for tetracycline?
   a) Take with Food
   b) Don't Take with Dairy or Iron Products
   c) Take with Milk
   d) For External Use Only

27) Which of the following is the correct method for reconstituting
    Ampicillin Suspension 125mg/5ml?
      a) Shake powder to loosen, then add entire contents of water
      b) Add entire contents of water and hit bottle against counter
      c) Shake powder to loosen, then add contents in divided portions
      d) Any of the above methods are acceptable

28) If a technician mixes 45gms of a HC 0.5% cream with 30 gms of a HC 1% cream,
    what is the resultant % in the total quantity of cream?
      a) 0.7%
      b) 0.6%
      c) 0.5%
      d) 0.4%

29) If a patient with hypertension asks the technician which cold remedy they
    recommend, the technician should:
      a) Tell the patient to call his/her doctor
      b) Tell the patient which cold remedy is suggested
      c) Ask the patient to wait to be counselled by the pharmacist
      d) Ask the patient to retake their blood pressure

30) An A ranking in the Orange Book indicates:
      a) that two drugs are bioequivalent
      b) that two drugs are in the same classification
      c) that two drugs are therapeutic equivalents
      d) that two drugs are therapeutic inequivalents

31) If a drug product expires 9/14, the drug expires:
      a) on the first day of the month
      b) on the last day of the month
      c) any time during the month
      d) on the 15th of the month

32) The phone number of a drug company would most likely be found in:
      a) Facts and Comparisons
      b) USP-DI
      c) Remington's Pharmaceutical Sciences
      d) Drug Topics "Red Book"

33) PCA pumps are used to administer which of the following medications?
   a) analgesics
   b) chemotherapuetic agents
   c) IV antibiotics
   d) insulin

34) A Drug Recall that results in death is considered a:
   a) Class I Recall
   b) Class II Recall
   c) Class A Recall
   d) Class B Recall

35) In which therapeutic class does the drug prochlorperazine belong?
   a) antihypertensive
   b) antibacterial
   c) antiviral
   d) antiemetic

36) "Net Profit" refers to:
   a) cash on hand
   b) cash after expenses
   c) cash prior to expenses
   d) zero profit

37) If a hazardous material is spilled, the technician should:
   a) clean the spill with isopropyl alcohol
   b) use absorbant towels to clean the spill
   c) clean the spill with a "Spill Kit"
   d) ignore the spill until after their shift, then clean it.

38) The size of the lumen of a needle is referred to as the:
   a) gauge
   b) length
   c) bevel tip
   d) bevel heel

39) In 1970, which piece of legislation was enacted?
   a) Hazardous Substance Act
   b) Occupational and Health Act
   c) Omnibus Budget Reconciliation Act
   d) Controlled Substance Act

40) How often is a federal inventory required for controlled substances?
    a) yearly
    b) every two years
    c) every three years
    d) only when the feds ask

41) A "HEPA FILTER" refers to:
    a) the filter found in a tranfer needle
    b) the filter used when withdrawing a drug from an ampule
    c) the filter found in the administration set of an IV
    d) the filter used in a laminar flow hood

42) Which of the following vitamins has antihemorrhagic properties?
    a) vitamin A
    b) Vitamin C
    c) Vitamin K
    d) Vitamin B

43) Which of the following drugs is available as a patch?
    a) nitroglycerin
    b) scopolamine
    c) fentanyl
    d) all the above

44) Which of the following drugs is a quinolone antibiotic?
    a) ciprofloxacin
    b) tetracycline
    c) penicillin
    d) erythromycin

45) If a prescription is written for penicillin VK 250 mg, ss tab po qid, how much drug will the patient receive each day?
    a) 0.125gm daily
    b) 0. 250gm daily
    c) 0. 375gm daily
    d) 0. 50 gm daily

46) A "Universal Claim Form" is used for:
    a) insurance fraud
    b) insurance billing
    c) insurance policies
    d) insurance theft

47) Which of the following drugs is a "NSAID"?
      a) acetaminophen
      b) aspirin
      c) ibuprofen
      d) codeine

48) Which drug must be mixed and stored in glass containers?
      a) NTG
      b) nitrofurantoin
      c) minoxidil
      d) clindamycin

49) What agent should be used to induce emesis?
      a) Compazine suppositories
      b) Tigan suppositories
      c) Syrup of Ipecac
      d) dilute HCl

50) The trade name for glyburide is:
      a) Diabinese
      b) Glucophage
      c) Glucotrol
      d) DiaBeta

51) An "ICD-9" code refers to:
      a) diagnosis
      b) drug strength
      c) manufacturer
      d) wholesaler

52) Which type of insulin may be added to an IV solution?
      a) NPH
      b) Lente
      c) SemiLente
      d) Regular

53) The generic name for Pamelor is:
      a) amitriptyline
      b) nortriptyline
      c) imipramine
      d) sertraline

54) If the directions read " ii gtts ad" the drug should be administered:
    a) in both eyes
    b) in the right eye
    c) in both ears
    d) in the right ear

55) Where should Domeboro tablets be stored?
    a) with the internal products
    b) in the refrigerator
    c) with the external products
    d) with the vaginal preparations

56) Which of the following drugs can be administered via aerosol?
    a) pentamidine
    b) chloroquine
    c) fluconazole
    d) miconazole

57) Which of the following DEA numbers is incorrect:
    a) AH 5847225
    b) AS 1993369
    c) BD 1654873
    d) all are correct DEA#s

58) The prefix "neuro" refers to:
    a) the lower extremities
    b) the brain
    c) the heart
    d) the spine

59) Theft of a Schedule II Controlled Substance from the dispensing area
    of a pharmacy would require notification to:
    a) DEA and State Board of Pharmacy
    b) DEA and local police authority
    c) DEA and FDA
    d) DEA only

60) What is the official storage temperature requirement for MS concentrate or
    oral solution?
    a) cold place
    b) cool place
    c) room temperature
    d) freezer

61) Federal statute requires the exact count of which medications?
    a) Ritalin and Percodan
    b) Ritalin and Vicodin
    c) Ritalin and Valium
    d) Ritalin and Darvon

62) "Grinding" of a substance into a fine powder is referred to as:
    a) geometric dilution
    b) levigation
    c) micturation
    d) trituration

63) Where should the pharmacy technician check for a possible
    incompatibility of two IV additives?
    a) American Drug Index
    b) Trissel's - Handbook of Injectable Drugs
    c) Remington's Pharmaceutical Sciences
    d) PDR

64) The generic name for " Persantine" is:
    a) alprostadil
    b) dipyridamole
    c) arbutamine
    d) pentoxifylline

65) DEA FORM 222 is required for the purchase of:
    a) Tylenol/codeine
    b) Vicodin
    c) Xanax
    d) Demerol

66) Cimetidine and Ranitidine are examples of:
    a) beta blockers
    b) NSAIDS
    c) H2 agonists
    d) H2 antagonists

67) Morphine would be classified as:
    a) a glycoside
    b) a benzodiazepine
    c) an opiate
    d) a quinolone

68) Proof of receipt of a C-IV controlled substance is:
     a) DEA Form 222
     b) wholesalers invoice
     c) narcotic inventory record
     d) end of day report

69) A third party reimbursement pays for a 14 day supply of medication.
   What quantity of medication should be dispensed for the following
   label directions: "i-ii tabs po q6-8 hours"
     a) 112
     b) 84
     c) 56
     d) 42

70) What type of syringe should be used in the preparation of a cytotoxic drug?
     a) glass
     b) plastic
     c) either glass or plastic
     d) a special syringe for cytotoxic use only

71) Gowns for preparation of hazardous materials close in the:
     a) back
     b) front
     c) side
     d) top

72) A special spill kit would be required for which of the following drugs?
     a) zidovudine
     b) famciclovir
     c) amphotericin B
     d) dactinomycin

73) Which of the following medications may cause heart palpitations?
     a) Nolvadex ID
     b) Claritin D
     c) Delta D
     d) Ascriptin A/D

74) Consider the following prescription:

Morphine SO4 10mg
Codeine PO4 10mg
Cherry Syrup 5ml
Ethyl Alcohol 5ml
qs water to make tbs

How many 20 mg morphine SO4 tabs would be required to make a pint of this mixture?
   a) 32
   b) 16
   c) 8
   d) 4

75) RX: Prednisone 5mg
         2 BID x 5 days

How many mgs will the patient take in a 48 hour period?
   a) 20
   b) 40
   c) 60
   d) 80

76) If a pharmacist makes 3 errors in 1500 prescriptions dispensed, what would be the % error rate?
   a) 0.2%
   b) 0.4%
   c) 0.6%
   d) 0.8%

77) What volume of glacial acetic acid is required to make 1/2 liter of a 0.25% glacial acetic acid solution?
   a) 5ml
   b) 10ml
   c) 2.5ml
   d) 1.25ml

78) One indication for the use of Ritalin is:
   a) mania
   b) hyperkinesis
   c) sleep disorders
   d) hepatitis C

182

79) A nosocomial infection is an infection classically acquired in a:
   a) outpatient clinic
   b) college dorm
   c) pet shop
   d) hospital

80) When federal and state law conflict, which law applies?
   a) state law
   b) federal law
   c) the more stringent law
   d) the more lenient law

81) The CDC regulates:
   a) dispensing of controlled substances
   b) disease control and prevention
   c) safety in the workplace
   d) drug safety

82) Mitomycin and plicamycin are two agents used to treat:
   a) cancer
   b) bacterial infection
   c) viral infection
   d) HIV

83) Which of the following diagnostic testing kits tests for blood glucose?
   a) Diastix
   b) Chemstrip UG
   c) Ketostix
   d) Chemstrip BG

84) If AWP for one hundred units of a drug is $45.92 and the pharmacy markup is 15%, what is the retail price for 30 units of this drug?
   a) $13.65
   b) $15.85
   c) $17.95
   d) $19.35

85) If the discount on a wholesaler invoice of $7300 is $219, the percent discount would be:
   a) 3%
   b) 6%
   c) 9%
   d) 12%

86) How should the pharmacy technician identify a drug product during a drug recall?
 a) lot#
 b) NDC
 c) expiration date
 d) bottle quantity

87) Which of the following medications is an antidepressant?
 a) gabapentin
 b) clozapine
 c) paroxetine
 d) omeprazole

88) If a patient profile lists granisetron and ondansetron as being administered together, this is an example of:
 a) therapeutic synergism
 b) therapeutic duplication
 c) therapeutic antagonism
 d) proper therapeutics

89) If the co-pay for a generic drug is $5.00 while for brand it's $10.00, what should the patient be charged for a drug in which the physician indicated "DAW"?
 a) $15.00
 b) $5.00
 c) $10.00
 d) $7.50

90) A hazardous drug must be prepared in a:
 a) vertical laminar flow hood
 b) horizontal laminar flow hood
 c) clean room
 d) anywhere is acceptable

91) Spansules and sequels are dosage forms for which route of drug administration?
 a) oral
 b) rectal
 c) sublingual
 d) buccal

92) If a patient is allergic to amoxicillin, there may be a cross allergy to which of the following drugs?
   a) tetracyline
   b) erythromycin
   c) Ceclor
   d) Nebcin

93) If the directions read " ii gtts ou bid x 7d, the medication is administered in:
   a) each ear
   b) each eye
   c) the right ear

94) Which part of the dispensing process must be documented in writing on a daily basis?
   a) inventory
   b) number of prescriptions filled
   c) controlled substance log
   d) net profit of prescriptions filled

95) "HEPA" stands for:
   a) a pharmacy organization
   b) a filter used on Laminar Flow Hoods
   c) a type of emulsifying agent
   d) the legislative act requiring childproof containers

96) If the AWP for a bottle of 100 Percocet is $55.56 with a 15% markup and a $6.00 dispensing fee, what would be the retail cost for 30 tablets?
   a) $20.55
   b) $21.66
   c) $22.77
   d) $25.16

97) If the cost of a Ventolin Inhaler is $21.05 and the pharmacy charges the patient $29.95, what is the markup rate for this medication?
   a) 42%
   b) 44%
   c) 46%
   d) 48%

98) Under Food, Drug and Cosmetic Act, which of the following information is not required on an outpatient dispensing label?
   a) name and address of the pharmacy
   b) date the prescription is filled or refilled
   c) name of the prescriber
   d) telephone number of the pharmacy

99) Hazardous drugs:
   a) must be stored in a vertical flow hood
   b) may be transported uncapped or unsealed
   c) may be prepared in a horizontal flow hood
   d) must contain a warning label affixed to the product

100) Which of the following drugs must be dispensed in its original glass container?
   a) Syrup of Ipecac
   b) NTG SL
   c) Tylenol/codeine Elixir
   d) Fosamax tablets

101) If a technician is unsure of who has supervisory authority, the technician should:
   a) ask the pharmacist on duty
   b) consult the organizational chart
   c) ask the CEO
   d) call the State Board of Pharmacy

102) Which of the following drugs is an H2 antagonist?
   a) Prevacid
   b) Protonix
   c) Axid
   d) Prilosec

103) Extemporaneous Compounding refers to:
   a) those drugs that are repackaged
   b) compounding of a drug not commercially available
   c) compounding your own recipe for a drug
   d) the use of a Class A Prescription Balance

104) Packing slips or invoices are acceptable as records for the transfer of which class of controlled substances?
- a) CI, CII, CIII, CIV, CV
- b) CI and CII only
- c) CII only
- d) CIII, CIV, CV only

105) A nurse calls the pharmacy asking for the proper dose of a drug. The pharmacy technician should:
- a) defer the question to the pharmacist
- b) check the dose in the PDR and relay this information to the nurse
- c) tell the nurse to ask the prescribing physician
- d) tell the nurse that you are unsure of the dose

106) The primary function of the P+T Committee is to:
- a) ensure that investigational drugs are not used in the institution
- b) ensure that the drugs used are the cheapest drugs possible
- c) ensure that all physicians have current DEA#'s
- d) ensure that all therapeutic agents used conform to USP-NF standards

107) Acetaminophen/codeine 15mg is commercially available as:
- a) Tylenol #1
- b) Tylenol #2
- c) Tylenol #3
- d) Tylenol #4

108) How many mls of a 2.5mg/5ml stock solution would be needed to prepare 3.5 liters of a 2mg/liter solution?
- a) 7mls
- b) 10mls
- c) 14mls
- d) 20mls

109) 97.5 mg is equivalent to how many grains?
- a) 1.5gr
- b) 2.0gr
- c) 2.5gr
- d) 3.0gr

110) Which of the following drugs requires an exact count for the federal
     biennial inventory?
     a) lorazepam
     b) propoxyphene
     c) meperidine
     d) phentermine

111) Enteral nutrition is administered:
     a) IV
     b) IM
     c) SC
     d) GI

112) If 1kg of an ointment contains 250gm of salicylic acid, what is the % strength
     of this ointment?
     a) 0.25%
     b) 2.5%
     c) 25%
     d) 250%

113) If a pharmacy stocks meds alphabetically by generic name, under which
     letter would generic Provera be found?
     a) L
     b) M
     c) N
     d) O

114) If morphine is infused at a rate of 0.8mg/hr, how many mls of morphine
     sulfate 2mg/ml would be needed for 12 hours of analgesia?
     a) 4.2 mls
     b) 4.4 mls
     c) 4.6 mls
     d) 4.8 mls

115) Which of the following drugs may be prepared in a horizontal laminar flow
     hood?
     a) dacarbazine
     b) vincristine
     c) gentamycin
     d) etoposide

116) Which drug reference has drugs listed by manufacturer?
  a) Fact and Comparisons
  b) Merck Index
  c) PDR
  d) Remington's Pharmaceutical Sciences

117) Which of the following drugs is not a benzodiazepine?
  a) Xanax
  b) Ambiem
  c) Versed
  d) Ativan

118) If the discount on a wholesaler invoice of $2750 is $302.50, what is the % discount of this invoice?
  a) 5%
  b) 7%
  c) 9%
  d) 11%

119) If the AWP for a drug is $67.90 and the drug retails for $74.99, what is the % markup for this drug?
  a) 5%
  b) 8%
  c) 10%
  d) 12%

120) Which of the following medications may not be taken together?
  a) tetracycline and ASA
  b) tetracycline and AlternaGel
  c) tetracycline and ranitidine
  d) tetracycline and Tylenol

121) If an investigational drug is discontinued by the physician, what must be done with the remaining drug?
  a) it should be destroyed
  b) it should be stored with the controlled substances
  c) it should be left to expire and discarded
  d) it should be returned to the manufacturer

122) The two parts of a needle are:
  a) the plunger and barrel
  b) the core and the gauge
  c) the hub and the shaft
  d) the hub and plunger

123) An adverse drug reaction should be reported to which of the following agencies?
    a) FDA
    b) DEA
    c) OSHA
    d) CDC

124) The combination of ethambutol, INH and vitamin B6 would most likely be used to treat:
    a) diabetes
    b) cancer
    c) hypertension
    d) TB

125) Which of the following drugs is an ACE Inhibitor?
    a) metoprolol
    b) lisinopril
    c) diltiazem
    d) clonidine

ANSWERS TO PRACTICE TEST #3

SEE NEXT PAGE

ANSWER KEY FOR PRACTICE TEST #3

1) a	26) b	51) a	76) a	101) b
2) c	27) c	52) d	77) d	102) c
3) c	28) a	53) b	78) b	103) b
4) b	29) c	54) d	79) d	104) d
5) d	30) c	55) c	80) c	105) a
6) a	31) b	56) a	81) b	106) d
7) b	32) d	57) c	82) a	107) b
8) a	33) a	58) b	83) d	108) c
9) a	34) a	59) b	84) b	109) a
10) d	35) d	60) c	85) a	110) c
11) d	36) b	61) a	86) a	111) d
12) c	37) c	62) d	87) c	112) c
13) b	38) a	63) b	88) b	113) b
14) d	39) d	64) b	89) c	114) d
15) a	40) b	65) d	90) a	115) c
16) c	41) d	66) d	91) a	116) c
17) b	42) c	67) c	92) c	117) b
18) a	43) d	68) b	93) b	118) d
19) d	44) a	69) a	94) c	119) c
20) b	45) d	70) c	95) b	120) b
21) d	46) b	71) a	96) d	121) d
22) b	47) c	72) d	97) a	122) c
23) c	48) a	73) b	98) d	123) a
24) d	49) c	74) b	99) d	124) d
25) d	50) d	75) b	100) b	125) b

PRACTICE EXAM #4

1) How must Nitroglycerin (NTG) be stored in an Emergency Crash Cart?
   - a) in a plastic bag
   - b) in a plastic vial
   - c) in its original glass bottle
   - d) any of the above is permitted

2) The grinding of a substance in a mortar and pestle is referred to as:
   - a) levigation
   - b) trituration
   - c) micturation
   - d) levitation

3) A pregnant pharmacy technician should avoid preparing:
   - a) cytotoxic drugs
   - b) IV antibiotics
   - c) TPN
   - d) all the above

4) The Policy and Procedures for Universal Precautions protects the pharmacy technician from exposure to:
   - a) airborne microorganisms
   - b) contamination by touch
   - c) fungal organisms
   - d) blood-borne pathogens

5) The primary benefit of automated medication dispensing systems is;
   - a) allow replenishment by nursing
   - b) track frequent adverse drug reactions
   - c) improved tracking and control of inventory
   - d) prevent diversion of controlled substances

6) Which committee is primarily involved with the formulary drug selection?
   - a) DUR Committee
   - b) P+T Committee
   - c) QA Committee
   - d) MD Committee

7) When a pharmacy technician calls a third party insurance company, which pharmacy ID number should they have available?
    a) DEA number
    b) pharmacy license number
    c) pharmacy provider number
    d) pharmacy insurance number

8) If the pharmacy technician notices that the medication storage refrigerator is at 53 degress F, they should:
    a) lower the temperature
    b) raise the temperature
    c) leave it alone
    d) make sure it's at room temperature

9) In a TPN, calcium chloride should not be mixed with which of the following salts?
    a) sulfate salts
    b) gluconate salts
    c) phosphate salts
    d) iron salts

10) Which of the following drugs is a Cox-2 Inhibitor?
    a) Cevalin
    b) Celexa
    c) Celestone
    d) Celebrex

11) Buccal tablets should be administered:
    a) vaginally
    b) in the cheek of the mouth
    c) rectally
    d) transdermally

12) How many mls of 95% ethyl alcohol must be mixed with water to make 1.5 liters of a 20% ethyl alcohol solution?
    a) 316ml of ethyl alcohol with 1184ml of water
    b) 573ml of ethyl alcohol with 927ml of water
    c) 624ml of ethyl alcohol with 876ml of water
    d) 787ml of ethyl alcohol with 713ml of water

13) What is the generic name for Cataflam?
   a) monoclofenac
   b) biclofenac
   c) triclofenac
   d) diclofenac

14) What is the final concentration when 15gms of codeine phosphate is dissolved in 1.5 liters of solution?
   a) 5mg/ml
   b) 10mg/ml
   c) 15mg/ml
   d) 20mg/ml

15) Nitrostat 1/200 gr is equivalent to how many milligrams?
   a) 0.22mg
   b) 0.33mg
   c) 0.66mg
   d) 0.88mg

16) Which of the following drugs treats Parkinson's Disease?
   a) levobunolol
   b) levodopa
   c) levocarnitine
   d) levofloxacin

17) To determine the generic equivalent rating of a drug, the pharmacy technician would consult which of the following textbooks?
   a) the Red Book
   b) the Green Book
   c) the Black Book
   d) the Orange Book

18) The CDC regulates:
   a) IV therapies
   b) waste disposal
   c) infection control
   d) disposal of Sharp's Containers

19) A physician prescribes Amoxil 375mg. Amoxil 250mg per 5ml is available. How many ml would be administered?
    a) 7.5ml
    b) 6.5ml
    c) 4.5ml
    d) 2.5ml

20) A prescription is written for an oral antibiotic to be taken as one teaspoonful every six hours. How long will a 200ml bottle last?
    a) 14 days
    b) 10 days
    c) 5 days
    d) 7 days

21) The dose of Cefamandole for children 3 months or older is 50-100mg/kg/day. What would be the daily dose range for a child who weighs 44 lbs?
    a) 0.3 - 1.0gm/day
    b) 0.6 - 1.2gm/day
    c) 1.0 - 2.0gm/day
    d) 2.2 - 4.4gm/day

22) When can a Schedule III or IV drug be refilled?
    a) monthly for up to one year
    b) when the supply runs out for up to one year
    c) a maximum of 5 times in a 6 month period
    d) as many refills indicated on the prescription

23) According to the Poison Prevention Packaging Act, who may waive childproof packaging?
    a) a physician
    b) a patient
    c) a pharmacist
    d) any of the above

24) Which of the following drugs requires a prescription?
    a) cimetidine
    b) sucralfate
    c) ranitidine
    d) famotidine

25) Which of the following drugs is commercially available as a transdermal patch?
    a) nitroglycerin
    b) scopolamine
    c) nicotine
    d) all the above

26) What is the required storage for Schedule III, IV and V controlled substances?
    a) in the safe with Schedule II narcotics
    b) in a locked closet
    c) dispersed among non-controlled drugs
    d) on a special shelf within the pharmacy

27) A third party reimbursement pays for a 30 day supply of medication. What quantity of medication should be dispensed for the following label directions: 1 and ½ tablets po QID?
    a) 180 tablets
    b) 135 tablets
    c) 105 tablets
    d) 95 tablets

28) Determine the flow rate of an IVPB containing 120ml of gentamicin, if the solution is to be infused over a 2 hour period and the administration set is calibrated to deliver 10 drops per ml.
    a) 20gtts/min
    b) 5gtts/min
    c) 7.5gtts/min
    d) 10gtts/min

29) The practice of perpetual inventory control occurs:
    a) on an annual basis
    b) when discrepancies are suspected
    c) on an ongoing basis
    d) on a quarterly basis

30) MAC pricing would be applicable to which type of product?
    a) chemotherapeutic agents
    b) multi-source generic drugs
    c) IV drugs
    d) single-source brand drugs

31) For proper aseptic technique, how long must hands be scrubbed with a suitable antimicrobial agent?
- a) until thoroughly cleansed
- b) 15 seconds
- c) 30 seconds
- d) 1 minute

32) EPA guidelines requires special disposal of:
- a) IV fluids
- b) IV antibiotics
- c) cytotoxic drugs
- d) all the above

33) What is the generic name for Provera?
- a) progesterone
- b) medroxyprogesterone
- c) norethindrone
- d) estradiol

34) Zidovudine is used to treat:
- a) herpes
- b) systemic fungal infections
- c) flu symptoms
- d) HIV

35) If the AWP for a drug is $77.90 and the drug retails for $84.99, what is the % markup for this drug?
- a) 8.32%
- b) 9.10%
- c) 10.44%
- d) 11.24%

36) The markup for a $38.75 vial of antibiotic is 19%. What is the retail price for this medication?
- a) $43.37
- b) $46.11
- c) $52.97
- d) $65.21

37) The cost of 500 tablets of ibuprofen 600mg is $82.28. If your pharmacy marks up the cost by 13% and adds a $2.35 dispensing fee, what would be the retail charge for 120 tablets?
    a) $23.57
    b) $24.66
    c) $26.54
    d) $27.46

38) Which of the following is required when dispensing a federally funded prescription?
    a) a federal discount
    b) dispense from a federal formulary
    c) always dispense a generic drug
    d) counselling on the proper use of the medication

39) A pharmacy technician may accept refill authorization from a physician only if:
    a) it is allowed by the State Board of Pharmacy
    b) it is authorized by the Director of Pharmacy
    c) it is authorized by the supervising pharmacist
    d) it is allowed by the local DEA office

40) Which of the following drugs is an aminoglycoside?
    a) ampicillin
    b) cefazolin
    c) tobramycin
    d) levofloxacin

41) Which auxiliary label would be appropriate when dispensing Tussionex?
    a) Take with food or milk
    b) Shake Well
    c) Take on an empty stomach
    d) Finish all medication dispensed

42) PCA pumps are used to administer which class of drugs?
    a) antibiotics
    b) chemotherapeutic agents
    c) IV fluids
    d) narcotic analgesics

43) What would a pharmacy technician look for during a nursing station inspection?
  a) initial use date of multi-dose vials
  b) expired medications
  c) proper storage of medications
  d) all the above

44) Which of the following drug regimens includes therapeutic duplication?
  a) Lanoxin, Normadyne and Vasotec
  b) Adalat, Accupril and Aldactone
  c) Lanoxin, Normodyne and Trandate
  d) Lasix, Inderal and Lanoxin

45) Which of the following auxiliary labels would be proper when dispensing the drug indomethacin?
  a) May cause drowsiness
  b) Take with food or milk
  c) Take on an empty stomach
  d) Finish all medication dispensed

46) How should epoetin alfa be stored?
  a) at room temperature
  b) in the freezer
  c) in the refrigerator
  d) there are no specific storage requirements for this drug

47) If 50 gms of a powder is repacked into 125 unit dose packages, how many milligrams will each package contain?
  a) 400 mgs
  b) 300 mgs
  c) 200 mgs
  d) 100 mgs

48) Lanoxin Injection is available in a concentration of 0.25mg per 1 ml. How many ml of the injection will be required for a 90 microgram dose?
  a) 0.2 ml
  b) 0.4ml
  c) 0.6ml
  d) 0.8ml

49) The dose of a drug is 0.25gr/kg of body weight. If the patient weighs 176 lbs, how many grams of the drug should the patient receive?
   a) 1.5 gms
   b) 1.4 gms
   c) 1.3 gms
   d) 1.2 gms

50) When preparing a cytotoxic drug in a hood, the pharmacy technician should be careful not to block the flow of air:
   a) horizontally
   b) diagonally
   c) vertically
   d) all of the above

51) Which of the following agents should be used to clean a Laminar Flow Hood?
   a) sterile water
   b) isopropyl alcohol
   c) betadine solution
   d) any of the above

52) CHF refers to a disease state affecting the:
   a) heart
   b) liver
   c) kidneys
   d) CNS

53) A syringe used to administer oral medications:
   a) may accept a needle
   b) must be made of glass
   c) must be made of plastic
   d) may not accept a needle

54) The last field of numbers of a drugs National Drug Code(NDC) indicates:
   a) the manufacturer of the drug
   b) indicates the drug product
   c) the size of the container
   d) the AWP of that drug

55) If 100 tablets of a drug contains 350mgs of active ingredient, how many grains of active ingredient would be contained in 250 tablets?
   a) 12.5gr
   b) 13.5gr
   c) 14.5gr
   d) 15.5gr

56) If epinephrine injection is available in a ratio concentration of 1:200, how would this concentration be expressed in mg/ml?
 a) 1mg/ml
 b) 2mg/ml
 c) 5mg/ml
 d) 10mg/ml

57) Which is the preferred dosage form of drug administration if a patient is vomiting?
 a) suppository
 b) tablet
 c) transdermal patch
 d) oral suspension

58) If the expiration date on a bottle of Ceclor tablets states 11/03, when does this medication expire?
 a) on the first day of the month indicated
 b) anytime during the month indicated
 c) on the 15th day of the month indicated
 d) on the last day of the month indicated

59) The initiation of Drug Recall is the responsibility of which organization?
 a) DEA
 b) NABP
 c) FDA
 d) OSHA

60) Which of the following drugs is used to treat a UTI?
 a) acyclovir
 b) ciprofloxacin
 c) gentamycin
 d) clindamycin

61) What should be the Pharmacy Technician's role in preventing diversion of controlled substances?
 a) ensure that all controlled substances are locked in a safe cabinet
 b) confront a patient thought to be abusing narcotics
 c) monitor a perpetual inventory of controlled substances
 d) conduct an inventory of all controlled substances monthly

62) Preparations containing hydrocodone belong to which Schedule of
    Controlled Substances?
    a) CIV
    b) CIII
    c) CII
    d) none of the above

63) The purpose of a Policy and Procedure Manual in a pharmacy is to:
    a) help in the training process
    b) make sure that tasks are performed properly
    c) ensure that tasks are performed in the same manner
    d) all of the above

64) The prescription label must contain:
    a) the date the prescription was written
    b) the date the prescription was filled
    c) the date the prescription was brought to the pharmacy
    d) the date the prescription was phoned in by the physician

65) A discount of $188 on a pharmacy invoice of $6250 represents what percent
    discount?
    a) 0.03%
    b) 0.3%
    c) 3%
    d) 33%

66) A prescription for a narcotic analgesic syrup is written to contain 10mg of
    codeine sulfate in each tablespoonful. How many 5 mg codeine sulfate
    tablets would be required to make 240ml of this syrup?
    a) 32 tablets
    b) 16 tablets
    c) 8 tablets
    d) 4 tablets

67) The AWP for 500 prednisone is $32.70. What would be the retail price for 100
    tablets if there is a 7% markup and a $3.50 dispensing fee?
    a) $7.50
    b) $8.50
    c) $9.50
    d) $10.50

202

68) Reconstituted amoxicillin is stable in the refrigerator for:
    a) 7 days
    b) 10 days
    c) 14 days
    d) 21 days

69) Plavix is similiar to which of the following drugs?
    a) Ticlid
    b) Tylenol
    c) Trental
    d) Coumadin

70) The label of a unit dose medication must include:
    a) NDC code
    b) manufacturing date
    c) date of prepackaging
    d) expiration date

71) The generic name for Persantine is:
    a) clopidogrel
    b) dipyridamole
    c) pentoxifylline
    d) tirofiban

72) The pharmacy technician wishes to find the compatibility of a drug in a
    parenteral solution. Which drug reference would provide this information?
    a) Remington's Pharmaceutical Sciences
    b) USP-DI
    c) AHFS Drug Information
    d) Handbook on Injectable Drugs

73) Mutamycin belongs to which of the following drug categories?
    a) antineoplastics
    b) aminoglycosides
    c) neuromuscular blockers
    d) beta blockers

74) If the computer flags a drug interaction, the pharmacy technician should:
    a) tell the patient that there is a drug interaction
    b) notify the physician of the interaction
    c) bring the drug interaction to the attention of the pharmacist
    d) override the computer and fill the prescription

75) DEA Form 222 is required when ordering which Controlled Substances?
 a) CII - CIV
 b) CII only
 c) CIII - CIV
 d) all Controlled Substances

76) When state and federal requirements conflict, which takes precedence?
 a) State law
 b) Federal law
 c) the most lenient law
 d) the most stringent law

77) Which type(s) of insulin may be added to an IV solution?
 a) Lente
 b) Regular
 c) NPH
 d) any of the above

78) What type of Drug Recall would be issued if a drug product caused temporary but reversible adverse effects to the patient?
 a) Class I Recall
 b) Class II Recall
 c) Class III Recall
 d) Class IV Recall

79) When pouring a liquid into a volumetric flask, the pharmacy technician should:
 a) use the top edges of the meniscus for a proper measure
 b) read the area between the top and bottom of the meniscus
 c) read the bottom of the meniscus for a proper measure
 d) any of the above methods is acceptable

80) If a technician wanted to investigate the compatibilities of two oral drugs, the best source of drug information would be:
 a) Drug Topics
 b) Remington's Pharmaeutical Sciences
 c) The Drug Index

81) Prior to dispensing an investigational drug to a nursing unit, the protocol must be approved by:
 a) P+T Committee
 b) Medical Board Committee
 c) Multidisciplinary Institutional Review Board
 d) JACHO

82) The AWP for a drug is $28.75 with a 12% discount from the wholesaler.
What would be the net cost of this drug?
a) $27.31
b) $25.30
c) $23.76
d) $22.13

83) Determine the flow rate of an IV if 50ml of drug is to be infused over 1 hour.
The administration set delivers 60gtts/ml?
a) 50gtts/min
b) 40 gtts/min
c) 25gtts/min
d) 10gtts/min

84) The pharmacy technician must prepare 1/2 liter of a D8W solution. How many
mls of D5W must be mixed with D10W to prepare this solution?
a) 100ml of D10W with 400ml of D5W
b) 400ml of D10W with 100ml of D5W
c) 200ml of D10W with 300ml of D5W
d) 300ml of D10W with 200ml of D5W

85) When the use of a drug leads to severe adverse effects or death, this recall is
categorized as a:
a) Class I Recall
b) Class II Recall
c) Class III Recall
d) Class IV Recall

86) An example of Biohazardous Waste would be:
a) needles used for drug preparation
b) an expired IV solution of a cephalosporin
c) an unused portion of a chemotherapeutic agent
d) all the above

87) MAC refers to the:
a) minimum allowable cost
b) maximum allowable cost
c) AWP price of a drug
d) HCFA price of a drug

88) If a prescription reads " ii gtts au qid', where would this medication be administered?
    a) in the right eye
    b) in both eyes
    c) in the left ear
    d) in both ears

89) Where are chemotherapeutic agents prepared?
    a) in a Biological Safety Cabinet
    b) in a Horizontal Laminar Flow Hood
    c) in a sterile area of the pharmacy
    d) anywhere is acceptable

90) Synagis is indicated for prevention of:
    a) HIV infections
    b) Herpes infection
    c) RSV infections
    d) allergic reactions

91) Synagis should be administered:
    a) weekly for 5-6 months
    b) monthly for 5-6 months
    c) every 6 months
    d) yearly

92) Synercid is a dual antibiotoc:
    a) available in IV dosage form only
    b) that should be reserved for vancomycin-resistant organisms
    c) that should be swirled not shaken when reconstituted
    d) all the above are true for this drug

93) If 30 grams of hydrocortisone 1% ointment are combined with 15 grams of a hydrocortisone 2.5% ointment, what is the resultant percentage concentration of hydrocortisone in the final product?
    a) 1.0%
    b) 1.5%
    c) 2.0%
    d) 2.5%

94) What is the final concentration when 12gms of codeine phosphate is dissolved in 1.5 liters of solution?
   a) 8mg/ml
   b) 10mg/ml
   c) 12mg/ml
   d) 16mg/ml

95) What is the ratio strength of a 20% solution ?
   a) 1:2
   b) 1:3
   c) 1:4
   d 1:5

96) Fentanyl trandermal patches are commercially available in which of the following strengths?
   a) 25, 50, 75 and 100mcg per day
   b) 10, 25, 50 and 100mcg per day
   c) 25, 50, 75 and 100mcg per hour
   d) 10, 25, 50 and 100mcg per hour

97) Net Profit is defined as:
   a) the revenue generated by the pharmacy
   b) the amount left over after all operating expenses are subtracted
   c) the measure of the percentage of profit
   d) the measure of inventory turnover

98) Prescriptions for controlled substances must contain the following information except:
   a) the physician's DEA number
   b) the patient's name and address
   c) the patient's age
   d) the physician's signature

99) The Omnibus Budget Reconciliation Act of 1990 requires pharmacists to perform which of the following functions?
   a) counselling
   b) drug regimen review
   c) drug utilization review
   d) all the above

100) How far within the laminar flow hood should sterile products be prepared?
- a) 12 inches
- b) 10 inches
- c) 8 inches
- d) 6 inches

101) If a medication is noted to be expired, the pharamacy technician should:
- a) discard the medication
- b) notify the DEA if it's a controlled substance
- c) adhere to the pharmacy's return procedure
- d) all the above are correct methods

102) If a patient is hypertensive, which of the following drugs are contraindicated?
- a) antihistamines
- b) nasal decongestants
- c) beta blockers
- d) diuretics

103) If a medication is prescribed "pc", this medication should be administered:
- a) after meals
- b) before meals
- c) with each meal
- d) with a bedtime snack

104) The purpose of Med Watch is to monitor:
- a) outcomes of therapy
- b) drug recalls
- c) diversion of controlled substances
- d) adverse reactions to drugs

105) Presciption drugs are also referred to as:
- a) investigational drugs
- b) legend drugs
- c) over-the-counter drugs
- d) new drugs

106) A liter of D5W contains how many grams of dextrose?
- a) 5 grams of dextrose
- b) 10 grams of dextrose
- c) 50 grams of dextrose
- d) 100 grams of dextrose

107) Normal Saline (NS) contains:
   a) 0.22% NaCl
   b) 0.45% NaCl
   c) 0.66% NaCl
   d) 0.9% NaCl

108) If a prescription reads " Cortisporin - ii gtts au q4h" which of the following products should be dispensed?
   a) ophthalmic ointment
   b) otic suspension
   c) ophthalmic solution
   d) otic solution

109) An inpatient hospital order is written for tobramycin 110mg in 50ml NS. How many ml of tobramycin 40mg/ml would be needed for this IVPB?
   a) 1.5ml
   b) 2.0ml
   c) 2.75ml
   d) 3.0ml

110) If 13 errors are made filling 260 prescriptions, what is the percentage error rate?
   a) 5%
   b) 0.5%
   c) 25%
   d) 0.25%

111) If the directions on a prescription read " ii tabs qod x30 days" and the AWP for that drug is $46.32/100, what is the cost of this prescription?
   a) $6.95
   b) $13.89
   c) $27.78
   d) $41.67

112) Consider the following patient profile:
    Vasotec 20mg po qd
    Depakote 250mg po tid
    Plavix 75mg po qd
    Ambien 5mg po qhs

Which drug would you suspect if the patient became hypotensive?
    a) Vasotec
    b) Depakote
    c) Plavix
    d) Ambien

113) Which drug information source would the pharmacy technician use to
    cross-reference a drug's generic, brand and chemical name?
    a) The Merck Index
    b) Facts and Comparisons
    c) The American Drug Index
    d) The Merck Manual

114) If a dozen gallons of distilled water cost $28.36, what would be the cost of
    5 gallons?
    a) $7.89
    b) $8.42
    c) $10.75
    d) $11.82

115) OSHA is the legislation that:
    a) protects the employer from being sued
    b) protects the worker within the workplace
    c) protects the employee from discrimination
    d) involves all of the above

116) A patient presents an empty vial of Percocet to be refilled. The pharmacy
    technician should:
    a) inform the patient that this medication is not refillable
    b) check the computer to see if there are any refills remaining
    c) call the physician for an authorized refill
    d) have the pharmacist authorize another refill

210

117) A prescription is written for Amoxil 375mg PO bid for 10 days. If the patient requests chewable tablets for their child, how many Amoxil 250mg Chewable tablets should be dispensed?
    a) 10
    b) 20
    c) 30
    d) 40

118) Which of the following medications may not be crushed?
    a) Inderal 10 mg tablets
    b) Depakote 250mg tablets
    c) Vasotec 5 mg tablets
    d) ASA 81mg tablets

119) The process whereby a drug is broken down in the liver is referred to as:
    a) absorption
    b) dissolution
    c) excretion
    d) metabolism

120) A pharmacy technician is asked to compound progesterone suppositories. Which drug reference would provide information on suppository bases?
    a) Fact's and Comparisons
    b) Drug Topics - The Red Book
    c) Remington's Pharmaceutical Sciences
    d) PDR

121) Which of the following dosage forms is used to mask an objectionable taste of a medication?
    a) tablets
    b) capsules
    c) IM injections
    d) SL tablets

122) Gloves, gowns, respirators and goggles should be worn when preparing:
    a) IV antibiotics
    b) TPN solutions
    c) progesterone suppositories
    d) chemotherapeutic agents

123) The directions for a prescription reads " ii tabs po tid pc and hs. How many doses should be dispensed for a 7 day supply?
   a) 56
   b) 42
   c) 34
   d) 21

124) Anabolic Steroids are categorized within which schedule of controlled substances?
   a) CI
   b) CII
   c) CIII
   d) CIV

125) Anabolic Steroid are chemically and pharmacologically related to which of the following drugs?
   a) progesterone
   b) estrogen
   c) testosterone
   d) all of the above

ANSWERS TO PRACTICE TEST #4

SEE NEXT PAGE

ANSWERS TO PRACTICE EXAM #4

1) c	26) c	51) b	76) d	101) c
2) b	27) a	52) a	77) b	102) b
3) a	28) d	53) d	78) b	103) a
4) d	29) c	54) c	79) c	104) d
5) c	30) b	55) b	80) a	105) b
6) b	31) a	56) c	81) c	106) c
7) c	32) c	57) a	82) b	107) d
8) a	33) b	58) d	83) a	108) b
9) c	34) d	59) c	84) d	109) c
10) d	35) b	60) b	85) a	110) a
11) b	36) b	61) c	86) c	111) b
12) a	37) b	62) b	87) b	112) a
13) d	38) d	63) d	88) d	113) c
14) b	39) a	64) b	89) a	114) d
15) b	40) c	65) c	90) c	115) b
16) b	41) b	66) a	91) b	116) a
17) d	42) d	67) d	92) d	117) c
18) c	43) d	68) c	93) b	118) b
19) a	44) c	69) a	94) a	119) d
20) b	45) b	70) b	95) d	120) c
21) c	46) c	71) b	96) c	121) b
22) c	47) a	72) d	97) b	122) d
23) b	48) b	73) a	98) c	123) a
24) b	49) c	74) c	99) d	124) c
25) d	50) c	75) b	100) d	125) c

PRACTICE EXAM # 5

1) When should a DEA Form 222 be completed?
   a) when a physician buys stock controlled-substances from the pharmacy
   b) when the pharmacy returns expired controllled drugs to the the wholesaler
   c) when the pharmacy returns controlled medications to the manufacturer
   d) all the above are correct

2) Which of the following drugs is an antiplatelet medication?
   a) ASA
   b) Plavix
   c) Aggrenox
   d) all the above are antiplatelets

3) What are some of the requirements for repackaging a unit dose?
   a) a log is maintained of repackaging activities
   b) no less than a six month expiration date is assigned
   c) the brand name of the drug must be used
   d) all the above are true

4) If a technician uses 350mg in D5W 500cc prepared with 500mg/20cc to stock. How much stock injection is added to create D5W ?
   a) 7ml
   b) 14ml
   c) 21ml
   d) 28ml

5) How often must a Laminar Flow Hood be certified?
   a) monthly
   b) quarterly
   c) every six months
   d) yearly

6) Of the following medications, which is a beta blocking agent?
   a) valsartan
   b) labetalol
   c) clonidine
   d) fosinopril

214

7) An average dose of Digoxin is considered to be?
   a) 0.25 mcg
   b) 0.25 mg
   c) 2.5 mcg
   d) 25 mg

8) What is the percentage mark up if a drug product is acquired for $27.76 and is resold for $39.95?
   a) 44%
   b) 33%
   c) 22%
   d) 11%

9) Policy and procedure manuals are developed to provide:
   a) safe and effective pharmacy operations
   b) consistency on how tasks are handled
   c) decisions on how situations are handled
   d) all the above

10) How many ml of a 70% dextrose solution are required to compound 200ml of a 20% dextrose solution?
   a) 27ml
   b) 37ml
   c) 47ml
   d) 57ml

11) Which drug is commonly implicated in having allergic cross-sensitivity with penicillin?
   a) gentamicin
   b) cefoperazone
   c) doxycycline
   d) sulfisoxazole

12) What special precaution is needed to ensure safety when compounding chemotherapeutic medications?
   a) use of a horizontal Laminar Flow Hood
   b) a gown that opens in the front in the event that the garment must be removed quickly
   c) use of a vertical Laminar Flow Hood
   d) syringes without Luer Lock tips

13) The diameter of the needle bore corresponds to:
     a) gauge
     b) length
     c) girth
     d) none of the above

14) Which drug is used in the management of diabetes?
     a) fluconazole
     b) captopril
     c) glipizide
     d) fluoxetine

15) How much MgS04 is required to prepare 500ml of 15% solution?
     a) 25gms
     b) 50gms
     c) 75gms
     d) 90gms

16) Clindamycin 300mg q6h is prepared from a solution of 75mg/5ml. How much volume is needed for 24hours?
     a) 20ml
     b) 40ml
     c) 60ml
     d) 80ml

17) The practice of placing newly received products behind old products in inventory is called?
     a) rotation
     b) replacement
     c) revolving inventory
     d) revolution

18) What do the first five digits of an NDC represent?
     a) product strength
     b) size of the packaging
     c) manufacturer
     d) none of the above

19) When using the drug sucralfate what is a normal dose?
     a) 0.5gm BID
     b) 1gm daily
     c) 1 gm QID AC
     d) 0.5gm TID PC

20) Where should Epoetin be stored?
    a) at room temperature
    b) in the refrigerator
    c) in the freezer
    d) in a warm area

21) Where would the technician find liquid Ativan?
    a) on the shelf with oral medications
    b) in the freezer
    c) on the shelf with the oral liquids
    d) in the refrigerator

22) When does a bottle of Xalatan Ophthalmic drops expire once it is opened?
    a) one week
    b) two weeks
    c) three weeks
    d) one month

23) The dose of Ticarcillin for an adult is 200mg/kg/day. What would be the dose for a 132lb adult?
    a) 1200mg
    b) 26.4gm
    c) 12gm
    d) 2640mg

24) What volume of MOM would you dispense to a patient if the dose is 2tbs BID PO for 16 days?
    a) 32 fluid ounces
    b) 16 fluid ounces
    c) a pint
    d) a gallon

25) What is the generic equivalent for Pamelor?
    a) amitriptyline hydrochloride
    b) amitriptyline pamoate
    c) nortriptyline hydrochloride
    d) nortriptyline pamoate

26) A severe allergic reaction to a drug is referred to as:
    a) prophylaxis
    b) anaphylaxis
    c) blephritis
    d) epistaxis

27) In what publication would the pharmacy technician find phone listings for a drug company?
    a) Merck Index
    b) Facts and Comparisons
    c) Remington's Pharmaceutical Sciences
    d) PDR

28) How many grams of magnesium sulfate is required to prepare a quart of a 50% magnesium sulfate suspension?
    a) 4.73gm
    b) 47.3gm
    c) 473gm
    d) 4730gm

29) Vitamin D is necessary in the body to:
    a) ensure calcium absorption
    b) prevent night blindness
    c) for muscle strength
    d) all the above

30) The pharmacy technician should affix which auxiliary labels when dispensing a prescription for an inhaler?
    a) Take With Food or Milk
    b) Shake Well
    c) May Cause Drowsiness
    d) all the above

31) How often should inventory of controlled substances be conducted?
    a) every year
    b) every 2 years
    c) every 3 years
    d) every 4 years

32) A 60kg elderly female patient must receive Dobutamine 72mg every day, infused over a four hour interval. Dobutamine is available in a concentration of 250mg/ml. What is the volume of Dobutamine in each daily cassette?
    a) 0.029ml
    b) 29ml
    c) 2.9ml
    d) 0.29ml

218

33) An infusion cassette of MgSo4 is 50mg/100ml PCA. In addition to the baseline dose 2mg/hr the patient receives bolus 1mg every 15 minutes. What is the total volume of solution the patient should receive in two hours?
   a) 24ml
   b) 20ml
   c) 16ml
   d) 12ml

34) Which of the following medications is considered a topical antifungal agent?
   a) acyclovir ointment
   b) clotrimazole cream
   c) azelaic acid cream
   d) gentamicin ointment

35) Cytotoxic agents are used in the treatment of what medical condition?
   a) CA
   b) HTN
   c) DM
   d) CHF

36) Which of the following agents is an antidepressant?
   a) Cogentin
   b) Ativan
   c) Lexapro
   d) Zyprexa

37) At what temperature should Humulin N be stored?
   a) between 36 and 46 degrees Fahrenheit
   b) between 46 and 59 degrees Fahrenheit
   c) between 59 and 86 degrees Fahrenheit
   d) between 86 and 104 degrees Fahrenheit

38) What is the resultant percentage strength when 10 pints of a 5% solution is diluted to 2 gallons?
   a) 6.2%
   b) 9.3%
   c) 12.4%
   d) 3.1%

39) What is the storage temperature for a Lorazepam injection?
    a) between 2 and 8 degrees Centigrade
    b) between -20 and -10 degrees Centigrade
    c) between 8 and 15 degrees Centigrade
    d) between 15 and 30 degrees Centigrade

40) Convert 98.6 degrees Fahrenheit to degrees celsius with this formula:
9C=5F-160
    a) 32 degrees Fahrenheit
    b) 34 degrees Fahrenheit
    c) 36 degrees Fahrenheit
    d) 37 degrees Fahrenheit

41) What is considered the best source of information for levels of responsibility among employees in a hospital pharmacy?
    a) Utilization Review Board
    b) patient education publications
    c) disaster procedure manual
    d) organizational chart

41) What is considered the best source of information for levels of responsibility among employees in a hospital pharmacy?
    a) Utilization Review Board
    b) patient education publications
    c) disaster procedure manual
    d) organizational chart

42) Which auxiliary label is needed when dispensing tetracycline?
    a) Take with food
    b) Do not take with dairy or iron products
    c) May cause drowsiness
    d) Take with plenty of water

43) "Direct" purchasing is from what source?
    a) wholesaler
    b) manufacturer
    c) pharmacy
    d) from the government

44) A 132lb patient is receiving Tobramycin 1.5mg/kg q8hours. How many mgs needs to be added to each IV piggyback?
   a) 30mg
   b) 60mg
   c) 90mg
   d) 120mg

45) What function does Allopurinol have in the body?
   a) inhibits uric acid production
   b) inhibits prostaglandin synthesis
   c) binds with opiate receptors in the CNS
   d) all the above

46) When preparing the surface of a laminar flow hood, which of the following disinfectants should be used?
   a) isopropyl alcohol
   b) hexachlorophine
   c) betadine
   d) any of the above are acceptable disinfectants

47) Which agent should be handled as "hazardous waste" if a spill occurs?
   a) heparin
   b) cyclophosphamide
   c) escitalopram
   d) olanzapine

48) Which of the following drugs is not a benzodiazepine?
   a) Ativan
   b) Xanax
   c) Restoril
   d) Atarax

49) Which of the following is considered an "anaphylactic" reaction?
   a) throat swelling
   b) hives
   c) difficulty breathing
   d) all the above

50) Which of the following drugs is an anticonvulsant?
   a) gabapentin
   b) diazepam
   c) lamotrigine
   d) all the above agents are anticonvulsants

51) Lovastatin is used to:
    a) raise triglycerides
    b) raise blood pressure
    c) lower blood pressure
    d) lower serum cholesterol

52) Which body organ does "arterial fibrillation" affect?
    a) nose
    b) bone
    c) heart
    d) stomach

53) An opiate overdose can cause which of the following conditions?
    a) diarrhea
    b) respiratory depression
    c) hypertension
    d) anxiety

54) Which ophthalmic product needs to be refrigerated to maintain potency?
    a) viroptic
    b) tobradex
    c) ciprofloxacin
    d) ofloxacin

55) A "drug interaction" can be described as:
    a) may be beneficial or harmful
    b) never results in death
    c) should always result in cessation of therapy
    d) are always flagged by the computer

56) Determine the flow rate required to deliver 250ml of an aminophylline drip
    to a 110 lb patient over a 2 hour period if the administration set is calibrated
    to deliver 60drops per ml?
    a) 60gtts/min
    b) 100gtts/min
    c) 125gtts/min
    d) 150gtts/min

57) Which of the following agents induces "emesis"?
    a) Compazine
    b) Thorazine
    c) Tegretol
    d) Ipecac

58) What is the cost of 90 tablets of quinidine sulfate 300mg, if 250 tabs cost $74.20?
    a) $23.42
    b) $26.71
    c) $28.93
    d) $30.04

59) When completing Form 222, the designee must:
    a) use blue ink only
    b) use red ink only
    c) never erase or alter any print
    d) print only

60) Which of the following medications provides dosage release in the intestinal tract and not in the stomach?
    a) enteric
    b) buccal
    c) film coated
    d) sublingual

61) Of the following flammable substances, which substance should be stored in a separate metal cabinet?
    a) acetone
    b) 95% ethyl alcohol
    c) elemental sodium
    d) all of the above

62) Determine the percentage concentration if 400ml of 80% solution is diluted to one liter.
    a) 32%
    b) 38%
    c) 42%
    d) 46%

63) Which of the following medications is an NSAID?
    a) acetaminophen
    b) APAP
    c) celecoxib
    d) fentanyl

64) Of the following medications, which is available only by prescription?
   a) omeprazole
   b) loperamide
   c) piroxicam
   d) clotrimazole

65) Simethicone is classified as an:
   a) antiflatulent
   b) antitussive
   c) antibiotic
   d) antiemetic

66) The pharmacy technician plays a key role in which quality improvement activity?
   a) therapeutic interchange
   b) adjusting insulin dosing
   c) collecting data for medication error reports
   d) selecting OTC preparations

67) A 132 lb patient receives 4mcg/kg of dopamine in a 1/2 hour interval. If the IV solution contains 800mcg of dopamine in 250ml D5W, what volume of IV dopamine should the patient receive?
   a) 50ml
   b) 75ml
   c) 10ml
   d) 25ml

68) How many mls of Tegretol 100mg/5ml is needed to administer a dose of 375mg of Tegretol?
   a) 15.25mls
   b) 16.5mls
   c) 17.35mls
   d) 18.75mls

69) How many milligrams are contained in 3 grains of desiccated thyroid?
   a) 160mgs
   b) 195mgs
   c) 210mgs
   d) 225mgs

70) Which of the following medications is an ophthalmic preparation?
    a) tobramycin
    b) gentamicin
    c) ciprofloxacin
    d) all the above

71) Once a product is dispensed, ownership of the prescription blank belongs to?
    a) insurer
    b) patient
    c) prescriber
    d) pharmacy

72) The requirement that a non formulary medication be covered only if the medication is approved by a third party payor is referred to as:
    a) capitation
    b) payor adjustment
    c) prior authorization
    d) claims recovery

73) Ordering medications directly from a manufacturer enables a pharmacy to:
    a) obtain the lowest pricing
    b) order smaller quantities
    c) reduce paperwork
    d) all the above

74) Which of the following organisms causes a viral infection?
    a) herpes simplex
    b) helicobacter pylori
    c) c. difficile
    d) candida albican

75) Which of the following can be safely compounded in a horizontal laminar flow hood?
    a) bleomycin
    b) mitomycin
    c) tobramycin
    d) doxorubicin

76) Which of the following is an over the counter analgesic?
    a) docusate
    b) ferrous sulfate
    c) diphenhydramine
    d) ketoprofen

77) Of the following medications, which can be obtained as a patch?
   a) fentanyl
   b) sumatriptan
   c) caffeine
   d) theophylline

78) What is the cost of 200gm of Bismuth Subnitrate USP. if two lbs costs $44.86?
   a) $7.38
   b) $8.64
   c) $9.88
   d) $20.19

79) When alcohol is used to disinfect a laminar flow hood, which concentration should be used?
   a) 10%
   b) 70%
   c) 50%
   d) 99%

80) From the following, select the correct DEA#:
   a) BD 5413242
   b) BH 7413242
   c) ED 8413242
   d) BB 9413242

81) When can a facsimile for a CII opioid analgesic serve as an original written prescription ?
   a) when the patient is out of the country
   b) in a certified hospice program
   c) in an investigational drug study
   d) a fax is never considered an original prescription

82) Which of the following is the generic equivalent to Anaprox DS?
   a) naproxen 550mg
   b) naproxen 500mg
   c)naproxen 220mg
   d) Anaprox DS has no generic equivalent
83) Cocaine belongs in which Schedule of controlled substances?
   a) Schedule IV
   b) Scehdule III
   c) Schedule II
   d) Schedule I

84) What amount of boric acid is needed to make 500gms of 4%(W/W) ointment?
    a) 5gms
    b) 10gms
    c) 15gms
    d) 20gms

85) Which of the following medications is a quinolone antibiotic?
    a) amoxicillin
    b) ciprofloxacin
    c) azithromycin
    d) erythromycin

86) What type of gown is required to be worn when preparing a hazardous drug in a biological safety cabinet?
    a) washable gown
    b) shortsleeve gown
    c) gown with loose fitting cuffs
    d) lint free low permeability fabric gown

87) How many gms of hydrocortisone powder are required to compound 16oz of 5% hydrocortisone cream?
    a) 18.6gms
    b) 22.7gms
    c) 25.8gms
    d) 29.9gms

88) If 10 ounces of a 20% solution is diluted with distilled water to one pint, what amount of active ingredient would be contained in 4 oz of the diluted solution?
    a) 60.6gms
    b) 45.5gms
    c) 15.2gms
    d) 36.8gms

89) Which of the following medications is cause for concern in patients allergic to ASA?
    a) bismuth subsalicylate
    b) lovastatin
    c) meclizine
    d) vitamin A

90) What volume is needed for a 24hour supply of 5% dextrose/0.45% NaCl at a
drip rate of 125ml/hr?
  a) 4 liters
  b) 3 liters
  c) 2 liters
  d) 1 liter

91) Which organization is responsible for determining whether a facility meets
criteria for accreditation?
  a) JCAHO
  b) Food and Drug Administration
  c) Department of Health and Human Services
  d) PTEC

92) Which of the following drugs is a cardiovascular medication?
  a) phenytoin
  b) diazepam
  c) digoxin
  d) valproic acid

93) The prefixes Hemat and Hemo refer to:
  a) lung
  b) blood
  c) lung and blood
  d) none of the above

94) Which reference text should be consulted by the technician to check the
compatibility of two additives in an IV solution?
  a) Trissel's
  b) Orange book
  c) PDR
  d) Remington's

95) How many grams of sodium sulfacetamide powder are required to
compound the following prescription:

sodium sulfacetamide - 10%
Eucerin and Moisturel - aa qs ad 90gms
  a) 1gm
  b) 3gms
  c) 6gms
  d) 9gms

96) A pediatric dose of phenobarbital is 3-5mg/kg. What is the dose range
    for a 55 lb child?
        a) 21mg - 35mg
        b) 30mg - 50mg
        c) 75mg - 125mg
        d) 300mg - 500mg

97) A single dose of a drug that is prepackaged is referred to as:
        a) single dose
        b) unit dose
        c) solo dose
        d) lone dose

98) Which drug is classified as a federally controlled substance?
        a) zolpidem
        b) zaleplon
        c) triazolam
        d) all the above

99) How many 2.5ml doses of acetaminophen elixir, containing 160mg/5ml,
    are contained in a 4oz bottle of the elixir?
        a) 12 doses
        b) 24 doses
        c) 48 doses
        d) 96 doses

100) What is the total number of individual supplies that can be ordered on one
    DEA Form #222?
        a) 4 items
        b) 6 items
        c) 8 items
        d) 10 items

101) What is the brand name for cefotaxime sodium?
        a) Cefotan
        b) Claforan
        c) Cefzil
        d) Cefobid

102) Which of the folllowing drugs is used to treat CHF?
    a) dapsone
    b) bupropion
    c) enalapril
    d) venlafaxine

103) Which of the following agents is a narcotic analgesic?
    a) meclizine
    b) melatonin
    c) celecoxib
    d) meperidine

104) Heparin belongs to which of the following drug categories?
    a) anticoagulant
    b) antiemetic
    c) antilipidemic
    d) antiemetic

105) How many 500mg tabs are required to compound 60ml of bethanechol chloride in 2g/ml of suspension?
    a) 60 tablets
    b) 120 tablets
    c) 240 tablets
    d) 360 tablets

106) When Schedule II drugs are shipped from a wholesaler, what information must be written on the purchaser's copy of DEA Form 222?
    a) NDC number, quantity, date
    b) date and signature
    c) number and size of packages ordered
    d) all the above must be present on DEA Form #222

107) If 90gms of HC 2.5% cream is mixed with 60gms of 1% HC cream, what is the resultant percentage concentration of HC in this cream?
    a) 1.6%
    b) 1.7%
    c) 1.8%
    d) 1.9%

108) Hepatic function refers to which body system?
    a) heart
    b) kidney
    c) liver
    d) lungs

109) Consider the following compounded prescription:
   Hydrocortisone 1%
   Menthol 1%
   Camphor 1%
   Nutraderm Lotion 1 pint

How many grams of camphor are needed to compound this prescription?
   a) 4.4gms
   b) 4.7gms
   c) 4.9gms
   d) 5.1gms

110) A patient is to receive 50mg q12h of Mellaril Oral Concentrate 30mg/5ml. How many mls would be needed for each dose?
   a) 8.3mls
   b) 8.4mls
   c) 8.5mls
   d) 8.6mls

111) In which schedule controlled substance does Phenobarbital belong?
   a) II
   b) III
   c) IV
   d) V

112) How long are Schedule II-IV drug records maintained for?
   a) 1 year
   b) 2 years
   c) 3 years
   d) 5 years

113) How many total milligrams are in a prescription for 30 tablets of thyroid 1 ½ gr?
   a) 2665mgs
   b) 2735mgs
   c) 2855mgs
   d) 2925mgs

114) DEA Form 222 is required to purchase acetaminophen in combination with which other ingredient?
   a) oxycodone
   b) codeine
   c) phenobarbital
   d) dextromethorphan

115) Which of the following best describes a "Negative Formulary"?
    a) list of medications approved for use
    b) medications carried by wholesalers and manufacturers
    c) list of medications that are not approved for use
    d) list of medications that are currently undergoing clinical study

116) Which computer based internet site is designed to allow for reporting of serious adverse drug reactions to the FDA?
    a) Drug Infonet
    b) Medwatch
    c) APhA site
    d) MERP

117) Which of the following drugs is a therapeutic duplication for Tenormin?
    a) Normodyne
    b) Capoten
    c) Catapres
    d) Vasotec

118) How much active ingredient is contained in 1oz of Anusol HC 2.5% cream?
    a) 75mgs
    b) 7.5gms
    c) 0.75gm
    d) 0.075gms

119) How should the technician dispose of used IV needles?
    a) special red plastic bags
    b) biohazardous waste bin
    c) trash bin
    d) Sharps Container

120) Which of the following agents need not be dispensed with special handling?
    a) doxorubicin
    b) methotrexate
    c) busulfan
    d) allopurinol

121) Which medication recall class states "use or exposure to will cause a severe health reaction or death"?
    a) Class I
    b) Class II
    c) Class III
    d) Class IV

122) Pharmacy technician support activities in an ambulatory anticoagulant
    clinic include?
    a) calculation of dose based on PT/INR's
    b) advise patient on diet and nonprescription medications
    c) inform the patient of possible drug interactions
    d) review of patients dosing calendar to note trends

123) Heparin belongs to which drug class?
    a) antiemetic
    b) anticonvulsive
    c) anticoagulant
    d) antitussive

124) How should the following directions be interpreted?
        "ii gtts au bid "
    a) instill 2 drops in each ear twice daily
    b) instill 2 drops in each eye twice daily
    c) instill 2 drops in the right ear twice daily
    d) instill 2 drops in the right eye twice daily

125) How often must a pharmacy do a complete inventory of
    controlled substances?
    a) every year
    b) every 2 years
    c) every 3 years
    d) every 4 years

ANSWERS TO PRACTICE TEST #5

SEE NEXT PAGE

ANSWERS TO PRACTICE EXAM #5

1) d	26) b	51) d	76) d	101) b
2) d	27) d	52) c	77) a	102) c
3) a	28) c	53) b	78) c	103) d
4) b	29) d	54) a	79) b	104) a
5) c	30) b	55) a	80) b	105) c
6) b	31) b	56) c	81) b	106) d
7) b	32) d	57) d	82) a	107) d
8) a	33) a	58) b	83) d	108) c
9) d	34) b	59) c	84) d	109) b
10) d	35) a	60) a	85) b	110) a
11) b	36) c	61) d	86) d	111) c
12) c	37) a	62) a	87) b	112) b
13) a	38) d	63) c	88) c	113) d
14) c	39) a	64) c	89) a	114) a
15) c	40) d	65) a	90) b	115) c
16) d	41) d	66) c	91) a	116) b
17) a	42) b	67) b	92) c	117) a
18) c	43) b	68) d	93) b	118) c
19) c	44) c	69) b	94) a	119) d
20) b	45) a	70) d	95) d	120) d
21) d	46) a	71) d	96) c	121) a
22) d	47) b	72) c	97) b	122) d
23) c	48) d	73) a	98) d	123) c
24) a	49) d	74) a	99) c	124) a
25) c	50) d	75) c	100) d	125) b

PRACTICE EXAM # 6

1) Which of the following is an example of a managed healthcare organization?
   a) PPI
   b) SOP
   c) MDHO
   d) HMO

2) Which drug administration route is the most convenient?
   a) PO
   b) IV
   c) IM
   d) SQ

3) EES (Erythromycin Ethyl succinate) is an antibiotic suspension that belongs to which of the following drug classifications?
   a) Cephalosporin
   b) Quinolone
   c) Macrolide
   d) Tetracycline

4) Included in the process of drug distribution, a pharmacy technician is responsible for all of the following EXCEPT:
   a) Controlling inventory levels
   b) Maintaining records
   c) Creating records
   d) Signing a DEA From # 222

5) Which of the following commercially available Tylenol w/ Codeine products is NOT a correct match?
   a) Tylenol #2- 15 mg of Codeine
   b) Tylenol #3- 30 mg of Codeine
   c) Tylenol #4- 60 mg of Codeine
   d) Tylenol #5- 75 mg of Codeine

6) Which one of the following anticonvulsants have both anticonvulsant and mood stabilizing properties?
   a) Depakote
   b) Dilantin
   c) Keppra
   d) Phenobarbital

7) Which of the following is NOT an example of automation?
   a) Baker cells
   b) Kirby-Lester counter
   c) Pyxis
   d) Sure-Med

8) The proper technique required when cleaning a Laminar Flow Hood is:
   a) Clean from the front of the hood to the back of the hood using 50% Isopropyl Alcohol
   b) Clean the hood from side to side using Sterile Water
   c) Clean from the back of the hood working towards the front of the hood using 70% Isopropyl Alcohol
   d) Clean the hood from back to front using Zephiran

9) How many 15ml doses are contained in 480ml of a medication?
   a) 0.03
   b) 32
   c) 30
   d) 3

10) How many doses are contained in 2.5 grams, if the dosage is 25mg?
    a) 1
    b) 10
    c) 100
    d) 200

11) Which Drug Recall class may cause temporary adverse health consequences?
    a) Class I
    b) Class II
    c) Class III
    d) Class IV

12) Which Federal Government Agency governs the classification of controlled substances with respect to "abuse potential"?
    a) DEA
    b) FDA
    c) CSA
    d) MDA

13) Which of the following is an itemized statement of all the merchandise on hand in a pharmacy setting?
- a) Inventory
- b) Turnover rate
- c) Overhead
- d) Gross sales

14) Which of the following is a fat soluble vitamin?
- a) Vitamin B-1
- b) Vitamin K
- c) Vitamin B-12
- d) Vitamin C

15) The FDA requires that generic versions of drugs have:
- a) A registered trade name
- b) A proprietary name
- c) A shortened version of its Brand Name
- d) The same active ingredients as the Brand Name

16) Roman numerals are expressed in Capital letters. Calculate the numeric translation for "XL":
- a) 40
- b) 50
- c) 4
- d) 5

17) How many grams of Ampicillin are in 10ml of a 500mg/1.5ml solution?
- a) 13g
- b) 1.3g
- c) 3.3g
- d) 333g

18) The FDA publishes a Drug Book that includes approved drug products, including therapeutic equivalence values. The title of this publication is:
- a) Red Book
- b) Orange Book
- c) Green Book
- d) Blue Book

19) Which of the following describes the rate and extent in which a drug is absorbed into the bloodstream?
   a) Metabolism
   b) Bioavailability
   c) Bioequivalence
   d) Distribution

20) The role of a pharmacy technician is to ensure the health and safety of a patient or customer. Which of the following duties may NOT be performed?
   a) Narcotic inventory
   b) Recommending an OTC product
   c) Preparing IV admixtures, aseptically
   d) Contacting an Insurance Company regarding coverage eligibility

21) According to the State Board of Pharmacy, every pharmacy must have specific compounding equipment for extemporaneous compounding. Which of the following balances is a requirement in the pharmacy setting?
   a) Class A Balance
   b) Class B Balance
   c) Bulk Balance
   d) Class AB Balance

22) What essential element is missing from the following prescription?
   Clarithromycin 1po qd x5 days
   a) Route
   b) Dosage strength
   c) Directions
   d) Duration of therapy

23) Concerning question #22, what function must be performed to ensure that this medication is taken correctly?
   a) Automatic stop order
   b) DAW authorization
   c) Automatic substitution order
   d) Negative Formulary

24) The process by which a drug is filtered by the liver is:
   a) Distribution
   b) First pass metabolism
   c) Elimination
   d) Pharmacokinetics

238

25) A physician writes an order for 5 million units of Penicillin. How many milliliters are needed if the available concentration of the drug is 500,000 units/ml?
    a) 1.0mg
    b) 10mg
    c) 10ml
    d) 100ml

26) Define the meaning of TPN:
    a) Total Patient Needs
    b) Three Parts Nutrition
    c) Treating Peripheral Nerves
    d) Total Parenteral Nutrition

27) How many milliliters of a 50% Dextrose solution are needed to prepare a 10g dose of Dextrose?
    a) 2ml
    b) 0.2ml
    c) 20ml
    d) 200ml

28) Which of the following drugs are used to treat GERD (Gastro- Esophageal Reflux Disease)?
    a) Lansoprazole
    b) Metronidazole
    c) Simethicone
    d) Gas X

29) The FDA is required to:
    a) Only monitor the drug prior to its approval
    b) Ensure that a drug is both safe and effective
    c) Approve the drug within 6 months
    d) Complete 2 out of 3 clinical trials before approval

30) How many ml's of 70% Dextrose must be mixed with 10% Dextrose to make one-half of a liter of 50% Dexrose?
    a) 122 ml of 70%
    b) 333ml of 70%
    c) 550 ml of 70%
    d) 188 ml of 70%

31) What is the meaning of a perpetual inventory?
   a) The recording of slow moving stock items
   b) Available merchandise on hand
   c) A constant count of items purchased and sold
   d) Accountability of stock on a monthly basis

32) Translate the following sig: i-ii gtts os q 12 h prn for blurred vision:
   a) 1-2 milliliters to right eye every 12 hours as needed
   b) 1-2 drops to right ear every 12 hours as needed
   c) 1-2 milliliters to left ear every 12 hours as needed
   d) 1-2 drops to left eye every 12 hours as needed

33) What is the generic equivalent for Celebrex?
   a) Cefotan
   b) Cefoxitin
   c) Celecoxib
   d) Cerebyx

34) Translate the Medical Abbreviation for DM:
   a) Diabetes Mellitus
   b) Double myopathy
   c) Diastolic murmur
   d) Digital method

35) An IV infusion of Methylprednisolone has been increased from 80mg to 110mg daily. What volume of Methylprednisolone 125mg/5ml would be needed for this new dose?
   a) 14ml
   b) 0.4ml
   c) 4.4ml
   d) 44ml

36) Listed below are examples of 3rd party payors, EXCEPT?
   a) Medicaid
   b) Medicare
   c) Insurance Companies
   d) PCA

37) The pharmacy budget is $74,000 for purchasing drugs. If the budget is set at $110,000 what % is allotted to purchase those drugs?
   a) 1.48%
   b) 74%
   c) 6.7%
   d) 67%

240

38) The NDC that is listed on a drug product label represents:
   a) New Drug Code
   b) New Disease Category
   c) National Drug Code
   d) Narcotic Drug Component

39) The number of times in which specific items are replaced during a finite period is called:
   a) Turnover rate
   b) Profit
   c) Inventory at cost
   d) Net

40) Rotating the inventory is an integral part in the day to day activities in the pharmacy setting. Which answer best describes why it is so important?
   a) It saves shelf space
   b) It allows for better lighting
   c) It insures the method of first in, first out
   d) It keeps the dust particles from getting on the labels

41) The Occupational Safety and Health Administration is responsible for all of the following EXCEPT:
   a) Maintaining a reporting system for injuries on the job
   b) Developing safety and health standards
   c) Conducting inspections
   d) Decreasing safety in the workplace

42) Before preparing a sterile IV admixture, the pharmacy technician must do all of the following procedures EXCEPT:
   a) Remove all jewelry
   b) Swab the needle shaft with alcohol
   c) Clean the IV flow hood with 70% alcohol
   d) Wash hands thoroughly

43) Which one of the following measuring devices affords a greater degree of accuracy when pouring liquids?
   a) A beaker
   b) A Cylindrical graduate
   c) A Conical graduate
   d) A volumetric flask

44) The NDC# is divided into 3 sets.   Identify these sets in chronological order:
   a) Manufacturer, dosage form and strength, quantity
   b) Dosage form, drug name, size
   c) Drug name, mg, bottle size
   d) Drug company, product size, mg

45) The Federal Government controls the use of drugs that can be potentially
   abusive. Of the five schedules, which has the highest abuse potential with no
   medicinal indications?
   a) I
   b) II
   c) I & II
   d) V

46) The smallest capsule size number is:
   a) 0
   b) 00
   c) 000
   d) 5

47) A pharmacy technician is asked to add 45Meq NaCl to an adult TPN.
   If the stock solution contains 2.5 Meq/2ml, how many ml's are
   required to complete this TPN?
   a) 36 ml
   b) 3.6 ml
   c) 0.36 ml
   d) 0.27 ml

48) Which of the following series of answers is correct regarding
   the 3 basic parts of a syringe?
   a) Calibration marks, hub, and tip
   b) Collar, barrel, and tip
   c) Barrel, plunger, and the piston
   d) Plunger, the calibrations, the luerlok tip

49) The DEA Form 222 is used to order CII substances. It must be signed by
   an authorized person. One copy is retained by the supplier, the 2nd copy is
   forwarded to the DEA. What is the disposition of the final copy?
   a) Is sent to the manufacturer
   b) Remains in the pharmacy
   c) Is sent to the CSA
   d) Is forwarded to the FDA

242

50) Which of the following is an example of an ACE inhibitor?
   a) Enalapril
   b) Propranolol
   c) Furosemide
   d) Albuterol

51) The three basic parts of the needle include:
   a) Hub, shaft, bevel edge
   b) Gauge, diameter, bore
   c) Collar, flange, tip
   d) The tip, the heel, the edge

52) The major source of contamination in a clean room is:
   a) The people in the room
   b) The keyboard on a computer
   c) The IV supplies
   d) The air circulation

53) Determine the flow rate to be used to infuse 750 mls of D5W over 8 hours. This set is calibrated to deliver 10 gtts/ml.
   a) 0.064 gtts/min
   b) 15.6 gtts/min
   c) 16.5 gtts/min
   d) 56 gtts/min

54) Epogen (erythropoietin) should be stored in a temperature not to exceed 46 degrees Fahrenheit. What is this temperature in Centigrade?
   a) 43.7 degrees C
   b) 23.4 degrees C
   c) 7.7 degrees C
   d) 9 degrees C

55) Medwatch is an organization that:
   a) Registers prescriptions
   b) Registers pharmacists
   c) Reviews medications prior to approval by FDA
   d) Encourages healthcare professionals to report an adverse drug reac

56) Meperdine (Demerol) belongs to which class of controlled substances?
a) CI
b) CII
c) CIII
d) CIV

57) Pharmacology is a term that describes which of the following?
a) The study of disease states
b) The identification of natural sources of drugs
c) The study of the combined effects of two drugs
d) The study of drugs and their actions pertaining to the body

58) Maintaining a patient's confidentiality was established by which of the following federal statutes?
a) CSA
b) HIPAA
c) CCS
d) DEA

59) What does the aconym ASHP stand for?
a) American School for Health Practicioners
b) American Society of Health Systems Pharmacists
c) Association of Sterile Hospital Products
d) American Standards for Healthcare Professionals

60) A PPI (Patient Package Insert) must be dispensed every time for which of the following drugs?
a) accutane
b) forane
c) butane
d) ethrane

61) Drugs are available by both prescription and non-prescription.
An example of a legend drug is:
a) An over the counter drug
b) An old drug
c) A drug that requires a prescription
d) A homeopathic remedy

62) Sulamyd Ophthalmic Solution would be instilled in the :
a) Nose
b) Eye
c) Ear
d) Mouth

63) The P&T committee includes all of the following healthcare
professionals EXCEPT:
    a) A registered pharmacist
    b) A registered nurse
    c) A registered dietician
    d) A clinical pharmacist

64) Which auxiliary label would be affixed to a vial containing
Cyclobenzaprine 10mg?
    a) May increase urine output
    b) May cause drowsiness
    c) May decrease appetite
    d) May cause excitability

65) Which of the following references would be used to investigate the
pharmacology and pharmacokinetics of a prescription medication?
    a) Merck Manual
    b) Facts and Comparisons
    c) USP-DI
    d) Goodman and Gilman

66) You have an ampule of Lanoxin that contains 500 mcg/ml.
What volume is needed to deliver a dose of 0.2MG?
    a) 8 ml
    b) 18 ml
    c) 0.8 ml
    d) 0.4 ml

67) The recommended practice for pharmacy personnel preparing cytotoxic
substances is to wear:
    a) Double gloves, gown, goggles
    b) Gloves, hairnet, shoe coverings
    c) Double gloves, hairnet, ventilator
    d) Gloves, mask, shoe coverings

68) When preparing an intravenous admixture the pharmacy technician must:
    a) Work 4 inches inside the hood
    b) Arrange supplies to the right side of the hood
    c) Work at least 6 inches inside the hood
    d) Arrange supplies to the left side of the hood

69) Which of the following DEA number is correct?
 a) AS2385638
 b) AB1234562
 c) AG3162213
 d) BB2311362

70) Which of the following is a collection of parenteral drugs containing stability, concentration, dosage and compatibility information?
 a) Trissels
 b) Remingtons Science
 c) USP-DI
 d) The Hypodermic Handbook

71) The disposal of cytotoxic material should be in a container that is labeled:
 a) Handle with care
 b) Confidential
 c) Biohazard
 d) Non-cytotoxic

72) Upon completion of an antibiotic IV admixture, the pharmacy technician must dispose the needle in:
 a) A sharps container
 b) A recycle bin
 c) A ziplocked bag
 d) The trash

73) Translate the medical abbreviation of COPD.
 a) Chronic Obstructive Pulmonary Disease
 b) Constant Original Pain Decongestant
 c) Continuous Output Per Deciliter
 d) Cardio-pulmonary Disease

74) The chemical element "Fe" stands for:
 a) Phosphorous
 b) Iron
 c) Sodium
 d) Potassium

75) Which of the following is an annual publication that provides prescription information, including pricing, on major pharmaceutical products?
 a) AHFS
 b) PDR
 c) PFR
 d) The Red Book

246

76) Interpret the following directions:

ss liter NS to run @ 125 ml/hr:

a) 1000 ml no sugar at 125 milliliters per hour
b) 500 ml Normal Saline at 125 milliliters per hour
c) 0.5 cc Normal Saline at 125 milliliters per hour
d) 1000 ml Normal Saline at 125 milliliters at bedtime

77) A child weighing 20 lbs has an order for an antibiotic that has a
recommended dosage range of 300-500 mg/kg/day in 3 divided doses.
What is the dosage range for one dose?
a) 4400 mg - 7333 mg
b) 909 mg - 1515 mg
c) 44 mg - 73 mg
d) 90 mg - 151 mg

78) Antihistamines are used in the treatment of allergies. Which of the following
is NOT an antihistamine?
a) Pseudoephedrine
b) Diphenhydramine
c) Claritin
d) Zyrtec

79) Which of the following pharmaceutical vehicles does NOT contain alcohol?
a) Tinctures
b) Elixirs
c) ETOH
d) Syrups

80) Which of the following answers best describes the indication
for Metformin?
a) Hypertension
b) Hyperglycemia
c) Hydronephrosis
d) Hyperproteinuria

81) Which of the following methods is considered to best reduce particle
size of a drug during extemporaneous compounding?
a) Geometric Dilution
b) Trituration
c) Flocculation
d) Levigation

82) Which organ is responsible for renal functions?
    a) Liver
    b) Pancreas
    c) Kidneys
    d) Heart

83) One of the components in a TPN is referred to as "fats." What is the medical terminology for "fat"?
    a) Lipids
    b) Cholesterol
    c) Triglycerides
    d) Acids

84) What is the most common cause of medications errors?
    a) Wrong patient
    b) Incorrect drug
    c) Poor legibility
    d) Overdose

85) Phosphates form insoluble precipitates when combined with which of the following elements?
    a) Calcium
    b) Magnesium
    c) Iron
    d) MVI

86) If a physician writes a prescription for a Proton Pump Inhibitor, which of the following drugs would NOT be considered?
    a) Aciphex
    b) Protonix
    c) Nexium
    d) Carafate

87) One cubic centimeter is equivalent to one:
    a) Millimeter
    b) Meter
    c) Milliliter
    d) Microliter

88) How many ml are required to make a prescription for one week of Maalox, dosed at 30 cc ac and hs?
 a) 4.8 ml
 b) 840 ml
 c) 720 ml
 d) 84 ml

89) How many milligrams are contained in one grain?
 a) 64.8 mg
 b) 30.6 mg
 c) 15.4 mg
 d) 1.2 mg

90) How tablespoonsfuls are contained in a pint and a half of Benadryl Elixir?
 a) 31 doses
 b) 47 doses
 c) 63 doses
 d) 72 doses

91) If a dose of Ampicillin is 5 ml q 8 hours for ten days, how many ounces will be needed to fill this entire prescription?
 a) 50 ounces
 b) 30 ounces
 c) 20 ounces
 d) 5 ounces

92) Of all the parenteral routes, which is the fastest?
 a) IM
 b) IV
 c) IT
 d) ID

93) What does the acronym SSRI stand for?
 a) Saunders Specific Reaction Index
 b) Selective Serotonin Reuptake Inhibitor
 c) Special Standards Regarding Insurance
 d) Selected Single Registered Inhalants

94) The Omnibus Budget Reconciliation Act:
 a) Requires authorization for prescription Insurance Coverage
 b) Regulates the pharmacy's budget
 c) Requires pharmacists to offer counseling to medicaid patients
 d) Reviews and reconciles third party payors

95) The air that circulates in a Vertical Flow Hood must:
   a) Flow from side to side
   b) Exhaust to the outside
   c) Flow downward onto the supplies
   d) Flow toward the pharmacy technician's face

96) Policy and Procedure Manuals are developed to provide:
   a) safe and effective pharmacy operations
   b) consistency on how tasks are handled
   c) decisions on how situations are handled
   d) all the above

97) What special precaution is needed to ensure safety when compounding chemotherapeutic medications?
   a) use of a horizontal Laminar Flow Hood
   b) a gown that opens in the front in the event that the garment must be removed quickly
   c) use of a vertical Laminar Flow Hood
   d) syringes without Luer Lock tips

98) An average dose of Digoxin considered to be?
   a) 0.25 mcg
   b) 0.25 mg
   c) 2.5 mcg
   d) 2.5 mg

99) Who is responsible for ordering investigational drugs?
   a) physician
   b) director of pharmacy services
   c) director of nursing
   d) only a Pharm. D

100) Which drug is classified as a federally controlled substance?
   a) zolpidem
   b) zaleplon
   c) triazolam
   d) all the above

ANSWERS TO PRACTICE TEST #6

SEE NEXT PAGE

ANSWERS TO PRACTICE EXAM #6

1) d	26) d	51) a	76) b
2) a	27) c	52) b	77) b
3) c	28) a	53) b	78) a
4) d	29) b	54) c	79) d
5) d	30) b	55) d	80) b
6) a	31) c	56) b	81) b
7) b	32) d	57) d	82) c
8) c	33) c	58) b	83) a
9) b	34) a	59) b	84) c
10) c	35) c	60) a	85) a
11) b	36) d	61) c	86) d
12) a	37) d	62) b	87) c
13) a	38) c	63) c	88) b
14) b	39) a	64) b	89) a
15) d	40) c	65) b	90) b
16) a	41) d	66) d	91) d
17) c	42) b	67) a	92) b
18) b	43) b	68) c	93) b
19) b	44) a	69) a	94) c
20) b	45) a	70) a	95) b
21) a	46) d	71) c	96) d
22) b	47) a	72) a	97) c
23) a	48) c	73) a	98) b
24) b	49) b	74) b	99) a
25) c	50) a	75) d	100) d

APPENDIX A - 2012 UPDATE:
TOP 200 DRUGS PRESCRIBED

The pharmacy technician is encouraged to create monographs of the top 200 drugs prescribed to ensure complete knowlegde of medications handled. Please refer to the example monogragh at the end of this section. The majority of drugs asked on the exam are asked in their generic names.

TRADE	GENERIC NAME	CLASSIFICATION
#1-10		
Lipitor	atorvastin	statin, high cholesterol
Nexium	esomeprazole	proton pump inhibitor
Plavix	clopidogrel	platelet inhibitor
Advair Discus	fluticasone/salmeterol	bronchodilator
Seroquel	quetiapine	atypical antipsychotic
Abilify	aripiprazole	atypical antipsychotic
Singulair	montelukast	antiasthmatic
Oxycontin	oxycodone	narcotic analgesic
Actos	pioglitazone	antidiabetic
Prevacid	lansoprazole	proton pump inhibitor
#11-20		
Cymbalta	duloxetine	antidepressant
Effexor XR	venlafaxine	antidepressant
Lexapro	escitalopram	antidepressant
Crestor	rosuvastatin	statin, high cholesterol
Zyprexa	olanzapine	antipsychotic
Valtrex	valacyclovir	antiviral
Flomax	tamsulosin	BPH
Lantus insulin	insulin glargine	antidiabetic
Lyrica	pregabalin	anticonvulsant
Celebrex	celecoxib	antiinflammatory
Levaquin	levofloxacin	antibacterial
#21-30		
Aricept	donepazil	Alzheimer's Disease
Spiriva	tiotropium	antiasthmatic
Diovan	valsartan	antihypertensive
Diovan HCT	valsartan/HCTZ	antihypertensive
Tricor	fenofibrate	antihyperlipidemia
Concerta	methylphenidate	CNS stimulant
Januvia	sitagliptin	oral hypoglycemic
Vytorin	ezetimibe/simvastatin	antihyperlipidemic
Adderall XR	amphetamine salts	CNS stimulant
Lovenox	enoxaparin	antithrombotic

TRADE	GENERIC NAME	CLASSIFICATION

#31-40

Atripla	three antivirals	antiviral/HIV
Zetia	ezetimibe	antihyperlipidemic
Aciphex	rabeprazole	proton pump inhibitor (PPI)
Ambien	zolpidem	hypnotic
Viagra	sildenafil	impotence agent
Topamax	topiramate	anticonvulsant
Lidoderm Patch	lidocaine topical	local anesthetic
ProAir HFA	albuterol	antiasthmatic inhaler
NovoLog insulin	insulin aspart	antidiabetic
Suboxone	buprenorphine/naloxone	narcotic analgesic

#41-50

Nasonex	mometasone	nasal steroid
Provigil	modafinil	CNS stimulant
Geodon	ziprasidone	atypical antipsychotic
Truvada	emtricitabine/tenofovir	antiviral/HIV
Lunesta	eszopiclone	hypnotic
Humalog insulin	insulin lispro	antidiabetic
Niaspan	niacin	antihyperlipidemic
Detrol LA	tolterodine	urinary antispasmodic
Yaz	drospirenone/estradiol	contraceptive

#51-60

Cozaar	losartan	antihypertensive
Namenda	memantine	Alzheimer's disease
Vyvanse	lisdexamfetamine	CNS stimulant
Tamiflu	oseltamivir	antiviral
Cialis	tadalafil	impotence agent
Arimidex	anastrozole	breast cancer
Enbrel	etanercept	antirheumatic
Flovent HFA	fluticasone	corticosteroid inhaler
Lantus insulin	glargine	antidiabetic
Combivent	albuterol/ipratropium	antiasthmatic

#61-70

Pulmicort	budesonide	antiasthmatic
Byetta	exenatide	antidiabetic
Benicar/HCT	olmesartan/HCTZ	antihypertensive
AndroGel	testosterone	anabolic steroid, topical
Prograf	tacrolimus	immunosuppressive
Hyzaar	losartan/HCTZ	antihypertensive
Benicar	olmesartan	antihypertensive
Premarin	conjugated estrogens	hormone replacement
Gleevec	imatinib	antineoplastic
Reyataz	atazanavir	antiviral/HIV

254

TRADE	GENERIC NAME	CLASSIFICATION
#71-80		
Boniva	ibandronate	osteoporosis
Strattera	atomoxetine	CNS stimulant
Lamictal	lamotrigine	anticonvulsant
Synthroid	levothyroxine	thyroid replacement
Humira Pen	adalimumab	antirheumatic
Solodyn	minocycline	antibiotic
Paxil	paroxetine	antidepressant
Chantix	varenicline	smoking cessation
Skelaxin	metaxalone	skeletal muscle relaxant
CellCept	mycophenolate	immunosuppressive
#81-90		
Evista	raloxifene	osteoporosis
Protonix	pantoprazole	proton pump inhibitor (PPI)
Xalatan	latanoprost	ophthalmic glaucoma
Actonel	risedronate	osteoporosis
Copaxone	glatiramer	multiple sclerosis (MS)
Femara	letrozole	antineoplastic hormone
Miraplex	pramipexole	antiparkinson
Avodart	dutasteride	BPH
Avandia	rosiglitazone	oral hypoglycemic
Humira	adalimumab	antirheumatic
#91-100		
NovoLog Mix 70/30	aspart protamine	antidiabetic insulin
Avapro	irbesartan	antihypertensive
Restasis	cyclosporin	anti-inflammatory (ophth)
Levemir insulin	detemir	antidiabetic
Avelox	moxifloxacin	antibiotic
Vesicare	solifenacin	urinary antispasmodic
Janumet	metformin/sitagliptin	antidiabetic
Sensipar	sinacalcet	hyperparathyroid
Aldara	imiquimod	topical anti-infective
Xopenex	levalbuterol	antiasthmatic
#101-110		
Seroquel XR	quetiapine	antipsychotic
Focalin XR	dexmethylphenidate	CNS stimulant
Renagel	sevelamer	chelating agent - Calcium
Avalide	irbesartan/HCTZ	antihypertensive
Keppra	levetiracetam	anticonvulsant
Actoplus Met	pioglitazone/metformin	antidiabetic, oral
Caduet	amlodipine/atorvastatin	antihyperlipidemic/HTN
Lotrel	amiodipine/benazepril	antihypertensive
NuvaRing	etonogestrel/estradiol	contraceptive
Norvir	ritonavir	antiviral/HIV

TRADE	GENERIC NAME	CLASSIFICATION
#111-120		
Kaletra	lopinavir/ritonavir	antiviral/HIV
Ventolin HFA	albuterol	antiasthmatic inhaler
Isentress	raltegravir	antiviral/HIV
Invega	paliperidone	antipsychotic
Prevacid	lansoprazole	proton pump inhibitor (PPI)
Risperdal	risperidone	antipsychotic
Depakote ER	divalproex	anticonvulsant
Avonex	interferon beta-1	multiple sclerosis (MS)
Doryx	doxycycline	antibiotic
Loestrin	norethindrone/estradiol	oral contraceptive
#121-130		
Forteo	teriparatide	osteoporosis
Pristiq	desvenlafaxine	antidepressant
Epzicom	abacavir/lamivudine	antiviral/HIV
Tarceva	erlotinib	antineoplastic
Proventil HFA	albuterol	antiasthmatic inhaler
Aggrenox	dipyridamole/ASA	antiplatelet
Lumigan	bimatoprost	antiglaucoma
Coreg CR	carvedilol	antihypertensive
Allegra-D	fexofenadine/pseudo	antihistamine
Welchol	colesevelam	antihyperlipidemic
#131-140		
Levitra	vardenafil	impotence agent
Kadian	morphine sulfate	narcotic analgesic
Ortho Tri-Cyclen Lo	norgestimate/estradiol	oral contraceptive
Xeloda	capecitabine	antineoplastic
Toprol XL	metoprolol	antihypertensive
Maxalt	rizatriptan	antimigrane agent
Nasacort AQ	triamcinolone	nasal steroid, topical
Zyvox	linezolid	antibiotic
Opana ER	oxymorphone	narcotic analgesic
Procrit	epoetin	anemia
#141-150		
Tussionex	hydrocodone/chlorphen	cough suppressant
Wellbutrin XL	bupropion	antidepressant
Exforge	valsartan/amlodipine	antihypertensive
Differin	adapalene	acne, topical
Humalog Mix	lispro/lispro protamine	antidiabetic, insulin
Combivir	lamivudine/zidovudine	antiviral/HIV
Vigamox	moxifloxacin	antibiotic, ophthalmic
Viread	tenofovir	antiviral/HIV
Trilipix	fenofibrate	antihyperlipidemic
Ciprodex Otic	ciprofloxacin/dexameth	antibiotic/anti-inflam

TRADE	GENERIC NAME	CLASSIFICATION
#151-160		
Actonel 150	risedronate	osteoporosis, monthly
Maxalt MLT	rizatriptan	migraine headaches
Duragesic Patch	fentanyl	narcotic analgesic
Asmanex	mometasone	antiasthmatic, inhaler
Relpax	eletriptan	migrane headaches
Entocort EC	budesonide	Crohn's disease
BenzaClin	clindamycin/BPO	acne, topical
Micardis	telmisartan	antihypertensive
Enablex	darifenacin	overactive bladder
Micardis HCT	telmisartan/HCTZ	antihypertensive, combo
#161-170		
Prezista	darunavir	antiviral/HIV
Revlimid	lenalidomide	antineoplastic
Travatan Z	travoprost	glaucoma, ophthalmic
Amitiza	lubiprostone	constipation, IBS
Alphagan	brimonidine	glaucoma, ophthalmic
Pegasys	peginterferon	hepatitsis C
Patanol	olopatadine	antihistamine, ophthalmic
Xyzal	levocetirizine	antihistamine
Fentora Bucal	fentanyl	narcotic analgesic
Catapres-TTS	clonidine	antihypertensive, patch
#171-180		
Clarinex	desloratadine	antihistamine
Avandamet	rosiglitazone/metformin	antidiabetic
Astelin	azelastine	antihistamine
Ultram ER	tramadol	analgesic
Zovirax	acyclovir	antiviral
Valcyte	vanganciclovir	antiviral
Uroxatral	afluzocin	BPH
Lialda	mesalamine	ulcerative colitis
Temodar	temozolomide	antineoplastic
Pentasa	mesalamine	ulcerative colitis
#181-190		
Allegra	fexofenadine	antihistamine
Propecia	finasteride	BPH
Vivelle-Dot	estradiol	estrogen patch
Zegerid	rabeprazole	proton pump inhibitor (PPI)
Premarin Vaginal	congugated estrogens	hormone replacement
Exelon Patch	rivastigmine	Alzheimer's disease
Prempro	cong. estrogens/medroxy	hormone replacement
Prandin	repaglinide	antidiabetic, oral
Imitrex	sumatriptan	antimigraine
Veramyst Nasal	fluticasone	corticosteroid

257

TRADE	GENERIC NAME	CLASSIFICATION
#191-200		
Taclonex	calcipotriene/betameth	psoriasis
Xopenex	levalbuterol	antiasthmatic
Duac	clindamycin/benzoyl	antiacne
Klor-Con	potassium chloride	K+ supplement
Xanax	alprazolam	antianxiety
Epipen Injection	epinephrine	allergic reactions
Avinza	morphine	narcotic analgesic
Atacand	candesartan	antihypertensive
Elmiron	pentosan	interstitial cystitis
Ativan	lorazepam	antianxiety

COMMONLY PRESCRIBED DRUGS
BY THERAPEUTIC CLASS

The pharmacy technician must know the generic name for each drug listed since the majority of drugs asked on the exam are in the generic names.

Acne Agents - Oral
Accutane

Acne Agents - Topical
Benzamycin
Cleocin T
Retin - A

Agents for Glaucoma
Alphagan   Timoptic
Trusopt   Xalatan

Agents for Gout
Zyloprim

Analgesics
Fioricet   Ultram
Fiorinal

Analgesics - Narcotics
MS Contin
Demerol   Percocet
Duragesic   Percodan
Fiorinal/Codeine Talwin NX
Lortab   Tylenol/Codeine
Vicodin

Antiasthmatic
Accolate
Singulair

Anti-inflammatory - Prostate
Flomax   Proscar

Anti-inflammatory - Steroids
Deltasone
Medrol
Prelone

Anti - Inflammatory - NSAIDS
Anaprox/DS Daypro   Relafen
Arthrotec   Lodine   Toradol
Cataflam   Motrin   Voltaren
Celebrex   Naprosyn

Antiallergy Agents
Beconase
Flonase
Nasocort
Nasonex
Rhinocort/AQ

Antianginals
Imdur
Nitro - Dur
Nitrostat

Antianxiety
Atarax
Ativan
Buspar
Valium
Xanax

Antiasthmatic - Bronchodilators
Atrovent   Serevent
Combivent   Theo-Dur
Maxair   Ventolin
Proventil

Antiasthmatic - Steroid
Flovent
Vanceril

Antibacterial - Topical
Bactroban

Antibiotic - Cephalosporin
Cefzil
Keflex
Omnicef
Suprax

Antibiotic - Macrolide
Biaxin   Zithromax
Erythromycin

Antibiotic - Penicillin
Amoxil   Veetids
Augmentin

Anticonvulsant
Depakote   Phenobarbital
Dilantin   Tegretol
Klonopin
Neurontin

Antidiabetic
Amaryl   Glucotrol
Avandia   Humulin
DiaBeta   Micronase
Glucophage   Rezulin

Antifungal - Topical
Lotrisone

Antifungal - Vaginal
Terazol

Antihistamine/Decongestant
Allegra-D
Zyrtec-D

Antibacterial - Antiprotozoal
Flagyl

Antibacterial - Sulfonamide
Bactrim/DS

Antibiotic - Carbacephem
Lorabid

Antibiotic - Fluoroquinolone
Cipro
Floxin
Levaquin

Antibiotic - Otic
Cortisporin Otic

Antibiotic - Tetracycline
Sumycin

Antidepressant
Desyrel   Remeron
Effexor   Serzone
Elavil   Tofranil
Paxil   Wellbutrin
Parnate   Zoloft
Prozac

Antifungal   **Antiviral**
Diflucan   Famvir
Lamisil   Valtrex
Nizoral   Zovirax

Antihistamine   **Antitussive**
Allegra   Tessalon
Phenergan   Tussionex
Zyrtec-D

Antihyperlipidemic

Lescol
Lipitor
Lopid
Mevacor
Pravachol
Zocor

Antimigraine Agent

Imitrex

Antipsychotic

Clozaril
Haldol
Risperdal
Seroquel
Zyprexa

Cardiovascular

Accupril (ACE-I)
Adalat (CCB)
Altace (ACE-I)
Avapro (Angio-A)
Calan/SR (CCB)
Capoten(ACE-I)
Cardizem(CCB)
Cardura(A-Block)
Catapres
Cozaar (Angio-A)
Diovan(Angio-A)
Hytrin(A-Block)
Hyzaar
Inderal (B-Block)
Isoptin (CCB)
Lopressor(B-Block)

Lotensin(ACE-I)
Monopril (ACE-I)
Norvasc (CCB)
Plendil (CCB)
Prinivil (ACE-I)
Procardia(CCB)
Tenorimin (B-Block)
Tiazac (CCB)
Toprol/XL(B-Blockl)
Vasotec(ACE-I)
Verelan(CCB)
Zestoretic
Zestril (ACE-I)
Ziac

Diuretics

Aldactone
Bumex
Dyazide
HCTZ

Lasix
Maxzide
Zaroxolyn

GI Antisecretory

Aciphex
Nexium
Prevacid
Prilosec

GI - H2 Antihistamine

Axid
Pepcid
Tagamet
Zantac

Antineoplastic

Nolvadex

Antivertigo

Antivert

Cardiovascular-Hemorheologic

Coumadin
Plavix
Pletal
Ticlid

Cardiovascular - Intropic

Lanoxin

CNS Stimulant

Adderall
Cylert
Dexedrine
Ritalin

Corticosteroid - Topical

Elocon
Lidex
Kenalog

Decongestant - Expectorant

Mucinex D

Erectile Dysfunction Agent
Cialis
Levitra
Viagra

Hormone - Combination
Prempro

Hormone - Estrogen
Estrace
Estraderm
Premarin

Hormone - Progestin
Cycrin
Provera

Hormone - Thyroid
Armour Thyroid
Levoxyl
Synthroid

Hypnotic
Ambien
Restoril
Sonata

Lower Respiratory Tract Agents
Tussionex

Narcotic Analgesics
Demerol
Duragesic
Lortab
Ms Contin
Oxycontin
Percocet
Percodan
Tylenol/codeine
Vicodin
Vicoprofen

Osteoporosis Agent
Evista
Fosamax
Miacalcin

Muscle Relaxants
Flexeril
Robaxin
Skelaxin
Soma

Ophthalmic Agents
Tobradex

Oral Contraceptives
Alesse
Demulen
Desogen
Loestrin/FE
Mircette
Necon
Ortho Tri-Cyclen
Ortho-Cept
Ortho-Cyclen
Ortho-Novum
Ovral/Lo
Tri-Levlen
Triphasil
Yasmin

Potassium Supplement
KCl

Smoking Cessation Aid
Zyban

Vitamin
Folic Acid

MONOGRAPH # _____

Generic name of drug: _____

Trade name and manufacturer: _____

(if multiple): _____

Therapeutic classification: _____
(basic mechanism of action)

_____

_____

Available dosage forms and strengths: _____

_____

_____

Special considerations: _____

_____

_____ _____

Appropriate auxiliary labels: _____

_____

_____

NOTE: The pharmacy technician is encouraged to create monographs of the top
medications prescribed. The example monograph style provides the
technician with basic information about drug products dispensed.

APPENDIX B: An Introduction to PBL

PROBLEM-BASED LEARNING (PBL)

This section contains Problem-Based Learning (PBL) type questions. Problem-Based Learning (PBL) is a learning process which uses a problem (i.e., a practice related scenario) to stimulate the acquisition of information, as well as, the application of the information acquired to the development of solutions.

The approach to identifying solutions to PBL based questions is the reasoning and decision-making process applied by the pharmacy technician to a specific case scenario. The technician is encouraged to search for the solution in the proper drug information source and to discuss possible solutions with fellow technicians and pharmacists.

An important prerequisite to the Problem-Based Learning approach is that the technician develop logical, organized reasoning and decision-making skills to identify and resolve problems. Many times different methods may be used to achieve similar goals, so there may be no absolute correct answer as is with standard multiple choice questions.

Try to form study groups between fellow technicians to discuss PBL problems and their decision-making processes.

I would like to thank my dear friend and colleague Roy Kemp, Jr., Director of Carver Career Center's Pharmacy Technology Program for submitting PBL questions and answers for problems #12 thru #15. Roy passed away in 1999 but his memory lives on through his work.

PROBLEM #1   **RX :   Meperidine 50mg**

 # 120

Sig: T PO TID for pain   Refill x2

a) Is this a proper prescription order or must this prescription be modified?

b) To which class of drugs does Meperidine belong?

c) Would the technician or pharmacist be responsible to explain any problems to the physician or the patient?

d) What is the maximum number of refills allowed for this medication?

e) Is this prescription to be administered as a "PRN" or a chronic medication?

f) What are the label requirements for this drug?

ANSWERS TO PROBLEM #1

a) The first problem with this prescription is that since Meperidine is a controlled substance, only a thirty day supply may be dispensed. With the medication being administered three times daily, only 90 tablets may be dispensed for a one month supply. A second problem is that the prescription states that this medication may be refilled two times. Since this medication is a Schedule II Controlled Substance, no refills are permitted to be dispensed.

b) This medication is a Schedule II narcotic analgesic used for the reduction of pain. Certain state regulations require the use of duplicate or triplicate copies of prescriptions for Schedule II substances. In this instance, a copy of the prescription must be forwarded to the appropriate state governmental agency, usually on a monthly basis. Other commonly dispensed Schedule II Controlled Substances include: codeine, Percodan, Percocet, oxycodone and morphine.

c) According to Federal Law, a pharmacy technician may not (1) transcribe a verbal medication order or (2) use professional judgement. For example, if a patient inquires to the technician as to which of two antacids they recommend, the technician must defer the question to the pharmacist since this involves professional judgement. As for the prescription above, the pharmacist must contact the physician to explain the prescribing discrepancies.

d) Since this is a Schedule II Controlled Substance, this prescription is non-refillable.

e) This prescription states that the medication is to be taken, by mouth, three times daily for pain. No where does this prescription indicate that the medication should be used as a "PRN" med. The label directions would read " Take one tablet by three times daily for pain."

NOTE: The National Certification Examinations ask questions relating to FEDERAL LAW only.

266

PROBLEM #2

A prescription is faxed by the physician to the pharmacy for the following:

Rx : ZITHROMAX SUSPENSION 200mg/5ml

Disp. 23ml

Sig: 100mg PO QD x10d for sinus infection

a) Briefly describe any irregularities with this prescription.

b) If the pharmacist is busy counseling a patient and your shift is over, write a short description of any problems in the communication log.

c) What is the legal status of a faxed or electronic version of a prescription order?

d) 12ml of distilled water must be added to reconstitute this medication. What type of volumetric graduate would be used to measure this liquid?

e) State the label directions and specify which auxiliary labels would be affixed to the prescription product?

f) To which category of drugs does Zithromax belong?

ANSWERS TO PROBLEM 2

a) The prescription states that the medication is to administered at a dose of 100mg daily for 10 days. The concentration of the suspension is 200mg per 5ml. Therefore to calculate the total volume of Zithromax suspension to be dispensed, the following proportion should be used: 200mg/5ml = 100mg/Xml   X = 2.5ml per dose. The medication is to be administered for 10 days so a total of 25ml is required for a 10 day supply. The physician incorrectly indicated that a quantity of 23ml should be dispensed. Since this formulation is available in 23ml or 30ml calibrated dispenser bottles, a 30ml quantity would be required to fill this prescription.

b) An example of a clear and complete communication in the log would be: " 2:30 PM - 11/16/11 - a prescription for patient Johnny Doe, age 4, is written incorrectly. The physician wants only 23ml to be dispensed for a 10 day supply. The correct volume required for a 10 day supply would be 25ml. Please document discrepancy on prescription".

c) Fax or computer-generated prescriptions are electronic variations of written prescriptions and maintain the same legal status as a written prescription. These orders are to be received and assessed in the same method as written prescriptions. The technician must remember that verbal medication orders may only be transcribed by a pharmacist.

d) Both conical and cylindrical graduates are available to the technician for accurate measurement of liquids. Cylindrical graduates are noted to be a bit more accurate than conical graduates. To measure 12mls of distilled water, the pharmacy technician should choose a cylindrical graduate whose total volume is as close as possible to the volume being measured. Measurements should always be made at eye level, reading the bottom most portion of the meniscus.

268

PROBLEM #3

The pharmacy technician receives a prescription from a patient and assesses that the prescription is complete and correct. When the technician returns to the computer to process the prescription, the computer has crashed and no further service will be available for the next five hours !!!

a) Must the dispensing process shut down or are there any other methods available to continue dispensing medications?

b) What would be the proper procedure for dispensing this prescription?

c) Describe the contents of the patient profile.

d) What type of documentation (log) would be required to be maintained?

e) Write a verbal communication that may be used to inform customers of an impending delay in filling prescriptions.

f) Describe any problems and possible solutions that may occur when the computer system comes back on-line.

ANSWERS TO PROBLEM #3

a) Computer prescription dispensing has become so much a part of pharmacy practice that when computer service is interrupted, pandemonium sometimes occurs. The pharmacy technician must be prepared for this event with an understanding of proper dispensing principles. In the interim while computer services are unavailable, a manual dispensing process must be initiated.

b) The major components of the dispensing process are the patient profile, label preparation, billing, prescription logging and medication preparation. Without computer function, each step of the process must be completed by hand with proper documentation. It is good pharmacy practice for all pharmacies to prepare for this inevitable event by having a written policy and procedure that addresses a manual backup dispensing procedure.

c) At the direction and under the supervision of the pharmacist, the pharmacy technician may interview the patient for vital information needed for the patient profile. This information should include: patient name, address and phone number, diagnosis, medication history and current usage, allergies, contraindications, special considerations and reimbursement of third party insurance information.

d) A "prescription log" must be maintained whenever a prescription is processed. In the computerized dispensing process, the prescription log is computer generated and must be reviewed and signed by the licensed pharmacist. The "prescription log" should include: date, patient's name, prescriber's name, and quantity of medication dispensed and identification of dispensing pharmacist.

e) Please understand that our computer dispensing system is down and that the prescription processing may take a little longer than usual. Would it be possible for you to return in a short while or may we deliver this prescription to your home?

PROBLEM #4

The pharmacy reviews the following compounded prescription and discusses the proper method of compounding with the pharmacist. After clarification of the compounding procedures, the pharmacist asks the technician to compound this prescription:

> Cherry Juice............................ 475ml
> Sucrose 100gm
> Alcohol 20ml
> Codeine PO4 .... 3mg/5ml
> Puried Water, qs t.o make .. 1000ml
> MAKE ONE PINT

a) Calculate the appropriate amount of each ingredient.

b) What is the correct method of compounding?

c) What type of balances would be used to weigh the sucrose and codeine?

d) The compounding cabinet contains methyl, ethyl, denatured and isopropyl alcohol. Which type of alcohol would be used for this prescription?

e) In which drug information source(s) would the technician find information about this compound?

f) Which auxiliary labels should be affixed to the prescription bottle?

ANSWERS TO PROBLEM #4

a) Cherry Juice - 475ml/1000ml = Xml/473ml   X = 224.6ml
    sucrose - 800gm/1000ml = Xgm/473ml   X = 378.4gm
    alcohol - 20ml/1000ml = Xml/473ml   X = 9.46ml
    codeine - 3mg/5ml = Xmg/473ml   X = 283.8mg
    purified water = enough to make 473ml

b) Dissolve the sucrose in the cherry syrup by heating it over a steam bath. Direct heat will cause the sucrose to turn brown (carmelization) and will give the syrup a burnt taste. Cool the mixture and remove any foam or floating solids. Dissolve the codeine phosphate in a minimum amount of purified water (2-3ml) and add to cherry syrup. Add the alcohol and sufficient purified water to make 473ml. The alcohol is present in this preparation to inhibit the growth of surface molds.

c) The codeine phosphate must be weighed out on a class A prescription balance. The minimum amount of ingredient that may be weighed is 120mg, with a maximum amount being 120gm. Since 378.4 gm of sucrose is to be weighed, a bulk balance would be used.

d) Methyl alcohol, methanol, must never be ingested since it can cause retinal damage and blindness. Isopropyl alcohol, rubbing alcohol is toxic upon ingestion and may not be used. Ethyl alcohol, ethanol, is suitable for ingestion and would be the proper alcohol for this antitussive cough preparation. Denatured alcohol is ethyl alcohol to which a denaturing agent has been added to make the ethanol unfit for ingestion.

e) Two drug information sources may be consulted for the proper method of compounding and for information on the physical properties of each ingredient. These would be the USP-NF and Remington's Pharmaceutical Sciences.

f) May Cause Drowsiness, Federal Transfer labeling and Shake Well auxiliary labels are necessary. Since the ethyl alcohol is less dense than the water, it will float on top of the preparation to retard mold growth in this highly concentrated sugar

PROBLEM #5

The pharmacy technician is asked to assist the pharmacist in compounding the following external preparation:

Zinc Oxide Ointment 20%
MAKE 6oz. of the ointment

a) If only a 25% ointment is available for compounding, how would you compound this ointment?

b) How many grains of active ingredient would be needed for this prescription?

c) What type of compounding equipment would be necessary to compounded this product?

d) Write a brief summary of your compounding technique so that others would know how you've compounded this prescription.

e) What are some common uses for the product and which dosage forms are commercially available?

ANSWERS TO PROBLEM #5

a) Since only a 25% zinc oxide ointment is available its concentration must be reduced with the addition of white ointment or white petrolatum. The method used to determine the quantities of each used would be "alligation alternate". In this problem the higher strength ointment is the 25% while the lower strength is 0%. With the desired strength being 20%, we calculate that 20 parts out of 25 total parts will be of the 25% ointment while 5 parts out of 25 total parts will be of the 0% ointment (white ointment/petrolatum). Therefore, to calculate the quantity of 25% ointment, the following proportion is used:

$$20 parts/25 parts = Xgm/180gm \quad X = 144gm \text{ of 25% zinc oxide ointment.}$$

To calculate the quantity of diluent or white ointment/petrolatum:

$$5 parts/25 parts = Xgm/180gm \quad X = 36gm \text{ of white ointment/petrolatum}$$

b) To calculate the amount of active ingredient, we calculate the total metric quantity and then convert to grains.

$$20\% = 20gm/100gm = Xgm/180gm \quad X = 36gm$$

To convert to grains, use the following conversion:

$$1gm/15.4gr = 36gm/Xgr$$
$$X = 554.4gr$$

c) The compounding equipment necessary would be a metal spatula, an ointment tile or paper, a prescription balance and a 6oz. ointment jar.

d) Weigh 144gm of the 25% ointment and 36gm of the white ointment/petrolatum. On an ointment tile or piece of compounding paper, place the 36gm of white ointment/petrolatum and add to this the 144gm of 25% ointment using geometric dilution. Geometric dilution is the method of adding equal amounts of different concentrations to ensure proper distribution of the active ingredient within the preparation. To the 36gm of white ointment/petrolatum add approximately 36gm of 25% ointment and levigate sufficiently until uniformly dispersed.
To this, add another equal quantity (70-75gm) of 15% ointment and levigate.

PROBLEM #6

Rx: Dilacor XR 240mg

 # 60

Sig: ii caps po daily with breakfast

a) Briefly describe the drug classification and the mechanism of action of this medication?

b) Name some indications of use for this medication.

c) List the brand and generic names for other medications in this class of drugs.

d) Is this a proper prescription order?

e) Describe the dosage form of the medication being dispensed?

f) What information should be conveyed by the pharmacist to the patient?

ANSWERS TO PROBLEM #6

a) Dilacor, diltiazem belongs to the group of drugs known as the Calcium Channel Blocking Agents. The mechanism of action of this category of drugs is the inhibition of calcium ions through the slow channels of the cardiac cells. This action may lead to the reduction of heart rate (chronotropism), a reduction in the strength of cardiac contractility (inotropism), reduction of peripheral vascular resistance and slowing of electrical conduction through the heart.

b) The indications of use are:

angina pectoris - where the oxygen supply to the heart is insufficient
hypertension - an increase in blood pressure
supraventricular tachycardia - excessive beating of the ventricle
atrial fibrillation and flutter - excessive beating of the atrium

c) (1) verapamil = Calan, Isoptin, Verelan (2) diltiazem = Cardizem, Dilacor XR
   (3) amlodipine = Norvasc   (4) felodipine = Plendil   (5) isradipine = DynaCirc
   (6) nicardipine = Cardene (7) nifedipine = Adalat, Procardia
   (8) nimodipine = Nimotop   (9) nisoldipine = Syscor   (10) nitrendipine = Baypress

   NOTE: Both Verelan and Cardene have IV dosage forms that is indicated for
         subarachnoid hemorrhage.

d) The directions for use states that two capsules should be taken by mouth daily with breakfast. Studies have shown that the rate of absorption is greater when administered with a high-fat breakfast. Therefore the manufacturer recommends administration of this medication on an empty stomach.

e) Dilacor XR capsules are extended-release capsules that should not be opened, chewed or crushed.

PROBLEM #7

> **RX: Altace 7.5mg**
> **#30**
> **Sig: i cap po qd x30 days**

a) Briefly describe any inconsistencies within this prescription.

b) To which class of drugs does Altace belong and what is it's mechanism of action?

c) List the brand and generic names for other drugs in this class of drugs.

d) Name some common drug interactions with Altace.

e) What drug information source(s) should be consulted for information on Altace's pharmacokinetics?

f) What information should the pharmacist convey to the patient?

ANSWERS TO PROBLEM #7

a) Altace, ramipril, is available as capsules only in the following strengths: 1.25mg, 2.5mg, 5mg, and 10mg. The prescription is written for 7.5mg of which no one dosage form is available. Therefore, this must be dispensed as two separate presciptions. One prescription would be for the 5mg capsules while the other would be for 2.5mg capsules.

b) Altace belongs to the category of drugs known as the angiotensin-converting enzyme inhibitors (ACE inhibitors). By inhibition of this enzyme, the conversion from angiotensin I to angiotensin II is reduced, and less angiotensin II, a potent vasoconstrictor, can exhibit it's hypertensive effects. These agents assume an important role in the treatment of hypertension and congestive heart failure.

c) Other ACE inhibitors are:
   benazepril (Lotensin), captopril (Capoten), enalapril (Vasotec)
   fosinopril (Monopril), lisinopril (Prinivil, Zestril), quinapril (Accupril)

d) 1) insulin, oral hypoglycemics - risk of hypoglycemia, especially at initiation of therapy. Monitor closely.
    2) lithium - increasd serum lithium levels. Monitor serum Li++ levels.
    3) potassium - increased risk of hyperkalemia. Monitor serum K+ closely.

e) Pharmacokinetics deals with drug absorption, distribution, metabolism and excretion of a drug. Some important drug information sources would be: Facts and Comparisons, AMA Drug Evaluations, or the PDR.

f) The pharmacist would want to alert the patient to possible swelling that might occur of the face, eyes, lips or tongue, especially after the first dose. The patient would also be counseled on the possibility of any light-headedness and to avoid abrubt discontinuation of this medication.

278

PROBLEM #8

RX: Brevibloc Injection - administer a loading dose of 500mcg/kg/ min. over 1 minute, then 50mcg/kg/min over 4 minutes as a maintenance dose

a) Discuss the drug classification and the mechanism of action of this medication.

b) Calculate the loading dose for an 89lb patient.

c) How would this IV solution be prepared?

d) Name some important indications for this drug.

e) List the brand and corresponding generic names for other drugs in this pharmacological category.

f) How would this drug be monitored?

ANSWERS TO PROBLEM #8

a) Brevibloc (esmolol) belongs to the class of drugs known as the beta adrenergic blocking agents. Activation of beta adrenergic receptors in the heart are responsible for increasing the speed and force of each contraction and also increases the electrical conductivity of the heart. By blocking these receptors in the heart, the rate and force of the heart can be slowed and made to beat less forcibly. Blocking beta receptors in the vasculature also causes a reduction of blood pressure.

b) To calculate loading dose, first change lbs to kg. 1kg/2.2lbs = Xkg/89lbs X = 40.45kg then calculate dose: 500mcg/1kg = Xmcg/40.45kg X = 20225mcg or 20.2mg of Brevibloc. This medication is commercially available in two concentrations: 2.5gm in a 10ml ampule and a 10ml single dose vial containing 100mg of the drug. Administration of Brevibloc is only in a final concentration of 10mg per ml.

c) Brevibloc should only be administered via syringe for the initial loading dose. Brevibloc is compatible in D5W, D5LR, D5R, D5 0.45%NaCl, D5 0.9%NaCl, Lactated Ringers, NaCl 0.45% and 0.9% Inj. It is not compatible with Sodium Bicarbonate 5% Injection or other drugs in the final solution.
Aseptically prepare a 10mg/ml solution by diluting two 2.5gm ampules in a 500ml container or one 2.5gm a pule in a 250ml container. This solution is stable at controlled room temperature for 24 hours.

> **NOTE:** Parenteral drug products must be inspected visually for particulate matter or discoloration prior to dispensing.

d) Brevibloc is indicated for rapid control of tachycardia and severe hypertensive episodes.

e) Other beta blocking agents include: (1) acebutolol - Sectral (2) atenolol - Tenormin (3) betaxolol - Kerlone (4) bisoprolol - Zebeta (5) carteolol - Cartrol (6) labetalol - Normodyne (7) metoprolol - Lopressor (8) nadolol - Corgard (9) penbutolol - Levatol (10) pindolol - Visken

f) This medication is monitored q4h and prior to administration by obtaining a pulse and blood pressure.

280

PROBLEM #9

The pharmacy technician receives the following medication orders:

Midamor tabs 5mg #30 Sig: 1 tab po qd

Micro-K caps 10mEq #30 Sig: 1 cap po qd

a) After assessing these orders, describe any inconsistencies with these orders.

b) List other brand and generic names of agents related to Midamor.

c) How are potassium levels monitored and what are some compliance problems?

d) What important patient information must be conveyed when dispensing this medication?

e) Name the indications for this group of medications?

ANSWERS TO PROBLEM #9

a) Midamor, amiloride is a potassium-sparing diuretic and would not require a potassium supplement. The physician would be notified that no potassium supplementation is needed for this diuretic. Other diuretics like the thiazides would require K+ supplementation.

b) Other potassium-sparing diuretics are:
   1) spironolactone - Aldactone, which is also available in combination with the thiazide diurectic HCTZ and is commercially known as Aldactazide.
   2) triamterene - Dyrenium is also available in combination with the thiazide diuretic HCTZ and is commercially known as Dyazide and Maxzide.

c) Levels of potassium in the blood, known as serum potassium, must be monitored on a regular basis. Normal serum potassium is 3.5 - 5.5 mEq/liter. Foods rich in potassium are bananas and oranges.

d) The patient should be counseled concerning the following:
   1) Since Midamor is a "water pill", diurectic that conserves potassium, no K+ supplementation will be needed and only one prescription will be dispensed.

   2) To arise slowly in the morning to avoid orthostatic hypotension, which is caused by the pooling of blood to the lower extremities and results in dizziness.

   3) To prevent hyperkalemia (increased seum K+), not to ingest excessive amounts of potassium rich foods, potassium containing salt substitutes or any potassium supplements.

e) Diuretics are indicated for hypertension and edema (swelling) associated with congestive heart failure (CHF).

f) The potassium-sparing diuretics interfere with sodium reabsorption at the distal sites in the renal tubule of the kidney.

PROBLEM #10

The pharmacy technician is asked to participate in the writing of a Policy and Procedure Manual for pharmacy services. You are asked to present an overview of the basic concepts of the Policy and Procedure process.

a) State the purpose of instituting policies and procedures in the pharmacy work place.

b) Discuss the important elements of composing a P+P manual.

c) Who is responsible for maintenance of the P+P manual?

d) List the major categories of the manual.

e) Discuss some problems associated with the policy and procedure process.

f) How should pharmacy P+P's be incorporated in the orientation process?

ANSWERS TO PROBLEM #10

a) A policy is a specific method or course of action while a procedure is a particular way of accomplishing that course. In pharmacy practice, to ensure that the same accurate and consistent outcome occurs, a set way of completing a particular task is set forth in the policy and procedure. They also help to standardize treatment of workers in the pharmacy setting. It serves as a:
   1) training manual for employees
   2) to minimize errors
   3) to eliminate waste
   4) to assist in job evaluation
   5) to serve as a legal document of activities, among others.

b) For the sake of consistency and to avoid confusion, policy and procedures should follow a specific template or format. Each P+P should be clearly titled and included in a table of contents so that it may be retrieved in an easy manner. Room should be allotted for approval and implementation dates along with notation of revision dates. Each P+P should be signed by at least two pharmacy personnel, one being the originator of the P+P while the other is usually an administrative representative. The body of the p+p must contain a formal statement of the policy and a detailed, logical step-by-step process of how the task is accomplished.

c) In the majority of institutional settings, the P+T (Pharmacy and Therapeutics) Committee is responsible for the approval of the P+P Manual. The Joint Commission on Accreditation of Healthcare Organizations (JCAHO) requires that the P+T Committee review and approve the policies and procedures of the department of pharmacy annually. All policies and procedures must comply with governmental (local, state and federal) laws and agencies.

d) The major categories of the P+P manual are:
   1) Organizational Aspects
   2) Personnel Issues
   3) Administrative Policies
   4) Professional Practice
   5) Facilities and Equipment

e) The most prominent problem associated with policies and procedures is enforcement. If P+P's are not adhered to then quality assurance becomes then quality assurance becomes the issue of concern.

f) Review of P+P's and standard procedures make up the majority of the orientation process.

PROBLEM #11

The pharmacy technician in charge of inventory is asked by the director of pharmacy to evaluate the effectiveness of current inventory practices.

a) What important indices would be used to evaluate cost effectiveness?

b) How is the turnover rate calculated?

c) How does a "formulary system" impact inventory costs?

d) Who are members of the P+T Committee?

e) What are some advantages of computerized inventory control ?

f) How does extemporaneous repacking effect inventory costs?

ANSWERS TO PROBLEM #11

a) Determining the turnover rate of drug inventory is an important method of measuring the overall effectiveness of inventory control. Source selection is also an essential step in assessing cost evaluation. Group purchasing, drug selection and substitution policies are all important contributing factors to materials management of pharmaceuticals.

b) The inventory turnover rate is calculated by dividing the total cost spent on purchasing pharmaceuticals for a one year period by the actual value of pharmacy inventory at any given time. This number indicates how many times in the course of one year the inventory has been replaced. The larger the number of inventory turnovers, the stronger the indication of an efficient inventory control program.

c) The selection of therapeutic agents that are available in the institutional pharmacy is governed by the Pharmacy and Therapeutics Committee. The official list of drugs available is called the "formulary", which must be reviewed and revised on an ongoing basis. The formulary helps reduce inventory costs by selecting the most cost effective therapeutic agent in a specific drug category rather than stocking each and every drug in that group. If a "non-formulary" drug is prescribed, the request must be reviewed by the appropriate process in order to decide if that drug will be dispensed. Strict adherence to the formulary allows for great reductions in pharmacy inventory costs.

d) The Pharmacy and Therapeutics Committee is chaired by a physician appointed by the medical director and its secretary is usually the director of pharmacy services. The committee is composed of representatives

e) Computer programs that monitor the purchasing, receiving and the dispensing process aid greatly in the evaluation of materials management. Perpetual inventory systems are utilized to indicate predetermined reorder points and monitor turnover rate accurately.

f) Repacking of bulk medications into unit-dose packages by automated packaging equipment is a valuable means of reducing inventory costs since the cost of buying unit-dosed medications is much greater than purchasing bulk products. The pharmacy technician must be knowledgable in this area with regard to record keeping and regulations governing repackaged medications.

PROBLEM #12

(written by Roy Kemp, Jr.)

The pharmacy technician is working in the IV area and receives the following order:

PT: Baby Boy Jones   Room 371-1   WT: 1.0 kg.

Ingredients	Amount Ordered
Amino Acids(5%)	1.5gm/kg
Dextrose(50%)	10%
NaCl (4meq/ml)	3meq/kg
KCl (2meq/ml)	1.5meq/kg
Mg SO4 (0.8meq/ml)	0.25meq/kg
Ca Gluconate(0.46meq/ml)	0.5meq/kg
Ped MVI	2ml/bag
Ped Trace Elements	0.9ml/bag
SWFI	qs
Volume = 110ml	Rate = 4.5ml/hr

a) Would this product be for sterile or nonsterile preparation?

b) What type of intravenous order is this?

c) What is TPN and what are other names used for this product?

d) What are some indications to receive Total Parenteral Nutrition?

e) How much of the dextrose(50%) injection must be added to this TPN?

ANSWERS TO PROBLEM #12

a) Since this medication will be for intravenous administration, it must be a sterile preparation. It must be prepared to minimize the potential for contamination with particulate matter, pyrogens, and bacteria. Non sterile compounding can be used for bulk and extemporaneous compounding.

b) This is a product called Total Parenteral Nutrition and in this case is for pediatric administration.

c) A patient may receive all of their nutritional requirements by intravenous administration. Some other names are: Total Nutrient Admixture, Hyperalimentation, IV Nutrition, Parenteral Nutrition, Hyperal, Central Hyperalimentation, etc.

d) Some patients who may need parenteral nutrition are those who are unable to eat, absorb or digest an adequate amount of nutrients in order to meet their current nutritional needs. Some examples are: bowel cancers, pancreatitis, Crohn's disease or other inflammatory bowel disease, perforated bowel, bowel surgery, trauma, leukemia, alaborption syndromes, AIDS, and others.

e) First, one must find the total amount of dextrose to be added: Total Volume = 110ml with the final concentration of dextrose being 10% = 11gm of dextrose. Using a 50% vial of dextrose, the technician must withdraw and inject 22ml of the 50% dextrose to achieve the 10% IV concentration.

PROBLEM #13   (written by Roy Kemp, Jr.)

Consider the following order:
1000ml D5W with 20meq K Cl + 2ml Berocca C @ 125ml/hr once daily.

a) Will the HEPA-filtered environment provided by the laminar airflow
   hood prevent contamination?

b) If the pharmacy technician used the laminar airflow hood and aseptic
   technique in preparation of this medication, what would be the
   most common contamination problem?

c) How long should the "hood" operate before this IV admixture is
   prepared?

d) What distance should the technician work within the laminar airflow
   hood and what is the zone of turbulence?

e) While preparing this IV admixture, the technician broke an ampule
   and a piece of glass perforated and lodged in the HEPA filter.
   What should the pharmacy technician do next?

ANSWERS TO QUESTION #13

a) No. Proper use of the laminar air flow hood is very important in the preparation of sterile products. Using strict aseptic technique is another important factor in IV admixture preparation procedures.

b)The laminar airflow hood will remove nearly all airborne contaminants. Therefore, touch will be left as the most common source of contamination of sterile products.

c) Actually, the LAH should operate continuously. If however the LAH is shut down, then employees should wait from 15 to 30 minutes for the LAH to purge room air before beginning sterile preparation. Manufacturer's recommendations should be consulted.

d) The technician should perform all aseptic manipulations at least six inches within the LAH. A zone of turbulence is created behind an object placed in the LAH. This will disturb the pattern of air being forced through the HEPA filter. Airflow should move on all sides of objects in the LAH. For example, if a vial is placed too close to the wall of LAH, the zone of turbulence could extend up to six times the diameter of this vial, extend outside the hood, and pull room air into the LAH.

e) The pharmacy technician should first report this accident to the supervising pharmacist. Nothing should be allowed to come in contact with HEPA filter. If damage is suspected, the LAH should be tested and recertified by qualified personnel.

PROBLEM #14

(written by Roy Kemp, Jr.)

The pharmacy technician is working in the clean room and receives the following order:

PT: John Doe, Jr   WT:70Kg.

Ingredients	Amout
Travasol 5.5% with electrolytes	1000ml
Dextrose 50% Inj	5%
KPO4 (4.4 meq K/ml)	3ml
Ca Gluconate (0.465 meq Ca/ml)	4 ml
MgSO4 (4.06 meq/ml)	2ml
MVI-12	1ml
Trace Elements	1ml
Liposyn	10%

Infusion Rate=30 min.
Administration set drop factor = 20
Infuse TPN every 12 hours

a) While entering this medication into Mr. Doe's drug profile, the technician notices that he is taking propranolol 40mg by mouth four times a day. What type of problem is this? What must the technician do?

b) After doing a review and analysis of this IV admixture, it was determined that their was a potential chemical incompatibility. What is this incompatibility dependent on? How can this incompatibility be overcome?

c) Upon further review it was decided that their was a pharmaceutical incompatibility in this preparation. What is this incompatibility and how can this be avoided?

d) At what rate would this preparation be administered in ml/hr and in drops/min ?

e) What resources would you use to check to see if these are the correct doses and concentrations?

ANSWERS TO PROBLEM #14

a) This could be an example of a therapeutic incompatibility. Labetalol and propranolol are sympatholytic drugs that oppose the action of the natural messengers, epinephrine and norepinephrine, at their receptor sites. Sometimes they are referred to as adrenergic antagonists, but more commonly they are called blockers. These two medications prevent another agent from acting at beta receptors and are called beta blockers. Beta blockers are used for the most part as antihypertensives. The first thing the pharmacy technician must do is to ask the pharmacist to certify that the drug order is entered correctly in the patient's profile. Second, this potential therapeutic incompatibility should be pointed out to the pharmacist. If these two drugs are to be administered concomitantly, the physician must be notified and asked to review these medication orders. The brand name for propranolol is Inderal. Labetalol is marketed under the brand names Trandate and Normodyne.

b) This IV admixture order presents the problem of a chemical incompatibility. The order of mixing calcium and phosphate may effect the compatibility of this solution, especially with increased concentrations of these electrolytes. Special care should be taken when adding these electrolytes. The phosphate should be added first and the solution should then be mixed or swirled. The calcium should be added to the bag last. Also, try to avoid adding magnesium directly after the phosphate. TPNs with high concentrations of calcium and phosphate should be inspected carefully. The precipitation of these two electrolytes can occur at a later time since they are not only concentration dependent, but also time and temperature dependent.

c) A usable and non-usable Total Parenteral Nutrition admixture must be distinguished by the physical appearance.
-Usable: No lipids - it should be a clear solution.
   Contains lipids - the emulsion should have a uniform milky appearance.
 -Unusable: No lipids-do NOT use if there is a white precipitate floating in the bag.
   Contains lipids- do NOT use if the layers have separated out. (Like vinegar and oil). Since the calcium and phosphate are concentration, time, and temperature dependent, this could create a possible pharmaceutical incompatibility. As stated earlier, the Liposyn should have a milky white appearance. If the calcium and phosphate form a precipitate, it may not be detected due to the milky, white color of the fat emulsion. Again, this possible pharmaceutical incompatibility should be pointed out to the pharmacist.

d) To calculate ml/hr, divide total number of hours of administration into total volume to be infused.

1000ml divided by 12 hours= 83.3 ml/hr
83.3 divided by 60 minutes = 1.39 ml/minute
1.4 ml/min. x 20 drops/ml. = 28 drops/minute

e) If you look up potassium phosphate in Facts and Comparisons you will find this solution will provide 3 mM phosphate and 4.4 meq potassium per ml. It also states that approximately 10 to 15 mM of phosphorous (equiv. to 310 to 465 mg elemental phosphorous) per liter of TPN is usually adequate to maintain normal serum phosphate. Also, in Facts and Comparisons you will see that a 10ml ampule of calcium gluconate contains 1gm of Calcium Gluconate or 90mg (4.5meq) of calcium. The adult dose is 0.5 to 2.0gm (5 to 20ml) as required or daily dose range is 1gm to 15gm. The adult dosage range of magnesium is 8 to 24 meq/day. Facts and Comparisons also gives you the electrolyte concentrations in the Travasol.

Their concentrations in meq/liter are:

Sodium	70
potassium	60
Magnesium	10
Chloride	70
Acetate	102
Phosphate	30mm/liter

Information about the incompatibilities can also be found in Lawrence A. Trissel's Handbook on Injectable Drugs. Under magnesium sulfate in Trissel's Handbook there is a section that deals with the incompatibilites of fat emulsions. There is also a complete explanation of the calcium and phosphate compatibility issue. Trissel's describes this as a conditional compatibility which is of a complex phenomenon. Lawrence A. Trissel also publishes a Pocket Guide To Injectable Drugs.

NOTES

NOTES